D1418648

CSA REVISION NOTES FOR THE
MRCGP

CSA REVISION NOTES FOR THE MRCGP

JENNIFER STANNETT
BSc (Hons), MBChB, nMRCGP, MRCPCH, DRCOG, DFSRH
GP in North London

Scion

ISBN 978 1 904842 86 6

First published in 2011

A CIP catalogue record for this book is available from the British Library.

Scion Publishing Limited
The Old Hayloft, Vantage Business Park, Bloxham Road, Banbury, Oxfordshire OX16 9UX
www.scionpublishing.com

Important Note from the Publisher
The information contained within this book was obtained by Scion Publishing Limited from sources believed by us to be reliable. However, while every effort has been made to ensure its accuracy, no responsibility for loss or injury whatsoever occasioned to any person acting or refraining from action as a result of information contained herein can be accepted by the authors or publishers.

Although every effort has been made to ensure that all owners of copyright material have been acknowledged in this publication, we would be pleased to acknowledge in subsequent reprints or editions any omissions brought to our attention.

Readers should remember that medicine is a constantly evolving science and while the authors and publishers have ensured that all dosages, applications and practices are based on current indications, there may be specific practices which differ between communities. You should always follow the guidelines laid down by the manufacturers of specific products and the relevant authorities in the country in which you are practising.

Typeset by Phoenix Photosetting, Chatham, Kent, UK
Printed by The Complete Product Company, Malmesbury, Wiltshire, UK

Contents

Preface

This book provides a summary of clinical cases which could be tested in the CSA exam, divided up into topics based on the MRCGP syllabus.

It aims to help prepare candidates for the CSA exam by providing a basic structure for consulting, focusing on the three key areas of data gathering, clinical management and interpersonal skills. The information is displayed in a concise manner in order to provide a quick reference guide for the candidate. It does not contain detailed clinical information. In the data gathering section, the most important aspects of history taking have been included and usually, but not always, cover history of the presenting complaint, past medical history, drug history, family history, and social history. Red flags have also been highlighted, where relevant, to act as a prompt to the reader to ask these important questions. Example questions have been included and these could be asked to explore the patient's ideas, concerns and expectations. I would also encourage you to think of your own alternative questions which you may also ask in the exam.

In the clinical management section I have included possible investigation and management options based on the latest UK guidelines. Not all options will be appropriate in every case, so it is important for the reader to consider each case individually.

Every case includes an explanation to the patient, which I hope will help the reader to think about how they would discuss each condition with the patient in jargon-free terms.

At the end of each case there is a role play scenario which can be practised in small groups or with a study partner. The information given to the doctor is similar to that which you will encounter in the CSA. The role player's brief should not be read by the doctor and so I suggest that the role player reads their information first and covers up the information (a Post-it note is ideal) before showing the doctor their information. Alternatively, the role player can read the brief to the doctor. The brief for the role player has deliberately been kept quite short in order to make it quick and easy to read, and the information in bold is that which should only be offered if asked about specifically by the doctor. Other clinical details can be added by the role player if necessary. The examination findings included in some cases can be given to the doctor if specifically requested, or alternatively they provide a good opportunity to practise these clinical examinations.

After completing each case in this book, it is important to reflect on how well you did in the role play scenario, and how you might improve your performance. It may be useful to ask the role player for their feedback. To make the most of the book, the role play scenarios should be practised under exam conditions. If working with a study partner, you could discuss each case in turn, teasing out various issues and then practising the scenarios again, trying out different techniques and consultation styles.

An explanation of the marking scheme and tips for success can be found in the first chapter, and the book concludes with appendices summarising the different clinical examinations which you could be expected to perform.

I would encourage readers to use this book like a workbook, gradually working through each clinical topic, and annotating it with your own aides-memoire to facilitate your learning. In the weeks leading up to the exam the book should be used in combination with lots of real patient consultations in the GP surgery. Together these will ensure that you go into the exam well prepared and confident.

Good luck!

Jennifer Stannett
December 2010

About the author

Jennifer Stannett gained a biomedical sciences degree from the University of Manchester before studying medicine at Leicester–Warwick Medical School. She spent two years working in paediatrics before completing vocational GP training in London. She is currently spending a year travelling the world and pursuing her interest in medical writing, before returning to full time general practice.

Acknowledgements

I would like to thank Paul Dakin, my former GP trainer, for his help, advice and inspiration to get involved in medical writing.

I would also like to thank my sister, Sarah, for her helpful comments and feedback, and my mum for her help with the book illustrations.

Most importantly thanks to my parents and fiancé Jerime for being so supportive over the years and helping me to reach my goals.

Abbreviations

A&E	Accident and emergency department		ECG	Electrocardiogram
ACE	Angiotension converting enzyme		ENT	Ear, nose and throat
ACR	Albumin creatinine ratio		ESR	Erythrocyte sedimentation rate
ADHD	Attention deficit hyperactivity disorder		FBC	Full blood count
AF	Atrial fibrillation		FEV1	Forced expiratory volume in 1 second
AFP	Alpha fetoprotein		FH	Family history
ALP	Alkaline phosphatase		FP10	Blank prescription
AMSE	Abbreviated mental state examination		FSH	Follicle stimulating hormone
			FVC	Forced vital capacity
BMI	Body mass index		GFR	Glomerular filtration rate
BNF	*British National Formulary*		GGT	Gamma glutamyl transferase
BP	Blood pressure		GI	Gastrointestinal
CBT	Cognitive behavioural therapy		GMC	General Medical Council
CF	Cystic fibrosis		GnRH	Gonadotrophin releasing hormone
CHD	Coronary heart disease		GORD	Gastro-oesophageal reflux disease
CK	Creatine kinase		GTN	Glyceryl trinitrate
CKD	Chronic kidney disease		GU	Genito-urinary
CKS	*Clinical Knowledge Summaries*		Hb	Haemoglobin
COCP	Combined oral contraceptive pill		HbA1C	Glycosylated haemoglobin
COPD	Chronic obstructive pulmonary disease		hCG	Human chorionic gonadotrophin
			HDL	High density lipoprotein
CPAP	Continuous positive airways pressure		HONK	Hyperosmolar non-ketosis
			HPC	History of presenting complaint
CRP	C-reactive protein		HRT	Hormone replacement therapy
CT	Computerised tomography		IBD	Inflammatory bowel disease
CVD	Cardiovascular disease		IBS	Irritable bowel syndrome
CVS	Cardiovascular system		ICE	Ideas, concerns and expectations
CXR	Chest X-ray		IDDM	Insulin-dependent diabetes mellitus
D&V	Diarrhoea and vomiting		IMB	Intermenstrual bleeding
DEXA	Dual energy X-ray absorptiometry		IRT	Immuno-reactive trypsinogen
DH	Drug history		IUCD	Intra-uterine contraceptive device
DKA	Diabetic ketoacidosis		IUD	Intra-uterine device
DM	Diabetes mellitus		IVDU	Intravenous drug user
DoH	Department of Health		LABA	Long acting beta agonist
DRE	Digital rectal examination		LDH	Lactate dehydrogenase
DSH	Deliberate self harm		LDL	Low density lipoprotein
DVLA	Driver and Vehicle Licensing Agency		LFTs	Liver function tests
			LMP	Last menstrual period
DVT	Deep vein thrombosis		LNG-IUS	Levonorgestrel intra-uterine system

LVF	Left ventricular failure	PR	*Per rectum* (rectally)
MC&S	Microscopy, culture and sensitivities	PRN	As required
		PSA	Prostate specific antigen
MED3	Fit for work certificate	PV	*Per vaginum* (vaginally)
MI	Myocardial infarction	PVD	Peripheral vascular disease
MMSE	Mini mental state examination	QDS	*Quarter die sumendus* (to be taken four times a day)
MRI	Magnetic resonance imaging		
MSU	Mid-stream urine	RA	Rheumatoid arthritis
NAAT	Nucleic acid amplification test	RhF	Rheumatoid factor
NAD	No abnormalities detected	RICE	Rest, ice, compression, elevation
NG	Naso-gastric	ROM	Range of movement
NICE	National Institute for Health and Clinical Excellence	RR	Respiratory rate
		RUQ	Right upper quadrant
NIDDM	Non-insulin dependent diabetes mellitus	SC	Sub-cutaneously
		SE	Side effect
NSAID	Non-steroidal anti-inflammatory drug	SH	Social history
		SHBG	Sex hormone binding globulin
NTDs	Neural tube defects	SL	Sublingual
OA	Osteoarthritis	SOB	Shortness of breath
OD	*Omni die* (once daily)	SSRI	Selective serotonin re-uptake inhibitor
O/E	On examination		
ON	*Omni nocte* (every night)	STI	Sexually transmitted infection
ONS	Office of National Statistics	SVT	Supraventricular tachycardia
OSAS	Obstructive sleep apnoea syndrome	T3	Triiodothyronine
		T4	Thyroxine
PALS	Patient Advice and Liaison Service	TDS	*Ter die sumendus* (to be taken three times a day)
PAPP-A	Pregnancy-associated plasma protein A		
		TFTs	Thyroid function tests
PCB	Post-coital bleeding	TIA	Transient ischaemic attack
PCOS	Polycystic ovarian syndrome	TOP	Termination of pregnancy
PE	Pulmonary embolus	TSH	Thyroid stimulating hormone
PEFR	Peak expiratory flow rate	U&Es	Urea and electrolytes
PHQ	Patient health questionnaire	UI	Urinary incontinence
PID	Pelvic inflammatory disease	UPSI	Unprotected sexual intercourse
PMB	Post-menopausal bleeding	USS	Ultrasound scan
PMR	Polymyalgia rheumatica	UTI	Urinary tract infection
PMS	Pre-menstrual syndrome	VT	Ventricular tachycardia
PO	*Per os* (orally)	VTE	Venous thromboembolism
PPI	Proton pump inhibitor	2WW	Two week wait

Introduction to the CSA examination

The CSA examination is both a clinical and a consulting skills examination. It is one of three parts of the new MRCGP, the other two being the Applied Knowledge Test (AKT) and the Workplace-Based Assessment (WPBA). The CSA is run three times a year at a purpose built examination centre in Croydon, and candidates can apply at any time during their GP registrar year.

The CSA examination is defined by the RCGP as '*An assessment of a doctor's ability to integrate and apply appropriate clinical, professional, communication and practical skills in general practice.*' The exam is based on the RCGP curriculum, and the cases are selected to include the wide spectrum found in everyday general practice.

Format of the examination

The CSA examination consists of 13 consultations, each of 10 minutes' duration. The circuit takes up to 3.5 hours to complete. All 13 cases will be marked.

Patients are played by trained role players. Examiners are selected, trained and monitored, and they sit in, observe and mark each candidate. There will be a different examiner for each case, with the examiner always remaining with the same role player and case for the entire duration.

Candidates stay in the same consulting room throughout the whole examination, the only exception being for a home visit or telephone consultation case.

Candidates are given case notes for each patient at the start of the examination. There are a few minutes to look through these notes prior to the examination starting. There are also 2 minutes between each case to look through these notes. The notes will include basic information about the patient, for example, name, age, relevant past medical history, current medication and social history.

A buzzer sounds to mark the start and end of each case, and there is a 15 minute break at the end of the seventh case.

A clinical examination may be required, and the examination you choose and how this is performed will be marked. You will not be expected to do any intimate examinations.

Prescriptions and sickness certificates can also be given to the role player, and these may be marked.

Candidates can offer patient information leaflets to patients, and can ask the patient to collect these from reception after the consultation. It is important to explain briefly the content of the information leaflet in order to gain credit for this.

If the consultation comes to a natural end before 10 minutes, the patient and examiner will get up and leave. Alternatively, if you haven't finished your consultation by the time the buzzer sounds at the end of 10 minutes, the patient and examiner will leave and you will not be marked for anything which happens after the buzzer.

Candidates are required to take a limited amount of equipment to the exam, including a BNF which can be used for reference during the examination. Further guidance on what to bring can be found on the RCGP website. Other equipment, for example growth charts, peak flow charts and an obstetric dial, is provided.

Marking scheme

The marking scheme was changed in September 2010. There is no longer a pass mark of eight out of 12 cases. The pass mark is set instead using a 'borderline group' method, which allows for day to day variability in the difficulty of case mixes. The examiner marks each case on three domains or areas:
- data gathering
- clinical management
- interpersonal skills

This creates an overall numerical mark for the case. Each domain carries the same number of marks. The marks for each case are added to create a final mark for all 13 cases. A pass mark will have been set by the combined judgements of the examiners for that day.

The following points highlight the key skills being assessed in each of the three domains.

Data gathering
- Organised and systematic in gathering information from history taking, examination and investigation
- Able to identify abnormal findings or results and recognise their implications
- Able to undertake physical examination competently, or use instruments proficiently

Clinical management
- Able to make an appropriate diagnosis
- Able to develop a management plan (including prescribing and referral) that is appropriate and in line with current best practice
- Able to demonstrate an awareness of management of risk and health promotion

Interpersonal skills

- Able to identify patient's agenda, health beliefs and preferences / makes use of verbal and non-verbal cues
- Identifies or uses appropriate psychological or social information to place the problem in context
- Develops a shared management plan or clarifies the role of doctor and patient
- Uses explanations that are relevant and understandable to the patient
- Shows sensitivity for the patient's feelings in all aspects of the consultation including physical examination

As well as marking the domain scores, the examiners will also mark each case separately using one of four possible grades:

- clear pass
- pass
- fail
- clear fail

Further details of these grade descriptors can be found on the RCGP website.

The table below lists the generic indicators used to compile the marking schedule, as noted by the RCGP on their website (www.rcgp.org.uk/docs/Exams_CSA_Generic domain_indicators_v9.doc). The website should be regularly checked for updated advice about the exam marking schemes.

Data gathering

Positive indicators	Negative indicators
• Clarifies the problem and nature of decision required • Uses an incremental approach, using time and accepting uncertainty • Gathers information from history taking, examination and investigation in a systematic and efficient manner. • Is appropriately selective in the choice of enquiries, examinations and investigations • Identifies abnormal findings or results and makes appropriate interpretations • Uses instruments appropriately and fluently • When using instruments or conducting physical examinations, performs actions in a rational sequence	• Makes immediate assumptions about the problem • Intervenes rather than using appropriate expectant management • Is disorganised/unsystematic in gathering information • Data gathering does not appear to be guided by the probabilities of disease. • Fails to identify abnormal data or correctly interpret them • Appears unsure of how to operate/use instruments • Appears disorganised/unsystematic in the application of the instruments or the conduct of physical examinations

Clinical management

Positive indicators	Negative indicators
• Recognises presentations of common physical, psychological and social problems • Makes plans that reflect the natural history of common problems • Offers appropriate and feasible management options • Management approaches reflect an appropriate assessment of risk • Makes appropriate prescribing decisions • Refers appropriately and co-ordinates care with other healthcare professionals • Manages risk effectively, safety netting appropriately • Simultaneously manages multiple health problems, both acute and chronic • Encourages improvement, rehabilitation, and, where appropriate, recovery. • Encourages the patient to participate in appropriate health promotion and disease prevention strategies	• Fails to consider common conditions in the differential diagnosis • Does not suggest how the problem might develop or resolve • Fails to make the patient aware of relative risks of different approaches • Decisions on whether/what to prescribe are inappropriate or idiosyncratic • Decisions on whether and where to refer are inappropriate • Follow-up arrangements are absent or disjointed • Fails to take account of related issues or of co-morbidity • Unable to construct a problem list and prioritise • Unable to enhance patient's health perceptions and coping strategies

Interpersonal skills

Positive indicators	Negative indicators
• Explores patient's agenda, health beliefs and preferences	• Does not inquire sufficiently about the patient's perspective/health understanding
• Appears alert to verbal and non-verbal cues	• Pays insufficient attention to the patient's verbal and nonverbal communication
• Explores the impact of the illness on the patient's life	• Fails to explore how the patient's life is affected by the problem
• Elicits psychological and social information to place the patient's problem in context	• Does not appreciate the impact of the patient's psychosocial context
• Works in partnership, finding common ground to develop a shared management plan	• Instructs the patient rather than seeking common ground
• Communicates risk effectively to patients	• Uses a rigid approach to consulting that fails to be sufficiently responsive to the patient's contribution
• Shows responsiveness to the patient's preferences, feelings and expectations	• Fails to empower the patient or encourage self-sufficiency
• Enhances patient autonomy	• Uses inappropriate (e.g. technical) language
• Provides explanations that are relevant and understandable to the patient	• Shows little visible interest/understanding, lacks warmth in voice/manner
• Responds to needs and concerns with interest and understanding	• Avoids taking responsibility for errors
• Has a positive attitude when dealing with problems, admits mistakes and shows commitment to improvement	• Does not show sufficient respect for others
• Backs own judgement appropriately	• Inappropriately influences patient interaction through own views/values
• Demonstrates respect for others	• Treats issues as problems rather than challenges
• Does not allow own views/values to inappropriately influence dialogue	• Displays inappropriate favour or prejudice
• Shows commitment to equality of care for all	• Is quick to judge
• Acts in an open, non-judgemental manner	• Appears patronising or inappropriately paternalistic
• Is cooperative and inclusive in approach	
• Conducts examinations with sensitivity for the patient's feelings, seeking consent where appropriate	• When conducting examinations, appears unprofessional and at risk of hurting or embarrassing the patient

After the CSA exam, you will be informed of your performance overall and your grades for the thirteen cases. This is the 'summative' part of the feedback. In addition, you will also receive 'formative' feedback, which is designed to help you to reflect on possible areas for improvement.

Formative feedback is given in relation to 16 areas of performance (see below). Not all of these are tested in every consultation although they will be tested across the assessment as a whole. Any area of performance identified as deficient by two or more examiners will be flagged in feedback as an area for improvement.

The following are the main feedback statements (see the RCGP website for further information).

Global

1. Disorganised/unstructured consultation.
2. Does not recognise the issues or priorities in the consultation (for example, the patient's problem, ethical dilemma, etc.).
3. Shows poor time management.

Data gathering

4. Does not identify abnormal findings or results or fails to recognise their implications.
5. Does not undertake physical examination competently, or use instruments proficiently.

Clinical management

6. Does not make the correct working diagnosis or identify an appropriate range of differential possibilities.
7. Does not develop a management plan (including prescribing and referral) reflecting knowledge of current best practice.
8. Does not make adequate arrangements for follow-up and safety netting.
9. Does not demonstrate an awareness of management of risk or make the patient aware of relative risks of different options.
10. Does not attempt to promote good health at opportune times in the consultation.

Interpersonal skills

11. Does not appear to develop rapport or show sensitivity for the patient's feelings.
12. Does not identify or explore information about patient's agenda, health beliefs and preferences.
13. Does not make adequate use of verbal and non-verbal cues. Poor active listening skills.
14. Does not identify or use appropriate psychological or social information to place the problem in context.
15. Does not develop a shared management plan, demonstrating an ability to work in partnership with the patient.
16. Does not use language and/or explanations that are relevant and understandable to the patient.

Tips for success

Below are a few tips to help you get through the CSA examination.

Preparing for the CSA

- Practise 10 minute consultations in readiness for the exam.
- Have a timed structure to your consultations, for example, 5 minutes for history taking, 2–3 minutes for examination, and 2–3 minutes for clinical management.

- Keep a logbook of the cases that you see in the GP surgery, and read up on clinical details you are unsure about.
- Try joint surgeries with your trainer and video your consultations, as this is a great way to get constructive feedback.
- Focus on practising cases you are less confident with; for example, a female registrar may not feel too confident with an erectile dysfunction case!
- Practise your examination skills on friends or family, especially those examinations that you might not perform frequently.
- Make sure you can interpret common results such as ECGs and spirometry.
- Try to attend a CSA course beforehand as it can be a great confidence booster.

On the exam day

- Arrive early.
- Remember to bring all the necessary equipment.
- Use the alcohol gel provided in between patients.
- Read through any information provided before each case commences and make notes if necessary.
- Make sure you cover all three domains within 10 minutes, as omission of any of these will result in a fail in that case.
- Be courteous and respectful towards the patients.
- Involve patients in decision making.
- Ensure that your explanations to patients are clear and jargon free.
- Drawing diagrams can be useful in aiding patient understanding.
- If you are referring a patient for further investigations or to secondary care, explain clearly what you intend to do.
- Check the patient's understanding and ask if they have any questions.
- If you lose your train of thought, try summarising the information you have already collected.
- If you feel one case didn't go so well, try to forget about it and regain your composure for future cases – remember you can still pass overall even if you fail some cases.
- Remember good communication skills and adopt a patient-centred approach.
- Try to remain calm.

General practice consultation

Telephone consultation

- In a climate of increasing targets and demand for access, telephone consultations are playing an increasingly important role in the delivery of healthcare by GPs.
- The scope of telephone consultations is wide ranging, and includes triage, management of acute and chronic problems, follow-up care and delivery of information.
- It is important to be aware of the limitations of telephone consultations. Telephone advice is not always appropriate, and they do not provide the non-verbal cues that make up around 50% of face to face consultations (*GPOnline*, 2008, *Consultation skills – telephone consultations*).
- Key skills in telephone consultations include active listening, frequent clarification and picking up cues such as changes in the tone of voice.

Framework for telephone consultations

Preparation
- Look through the patient's notes prior to the telephone call, familiarising yourself with their past medical history, medication history and recent consultations, etc.

Introduction
- Introduce yourself and ensure that you are speaking to the correct person to ensure confidentiality.
- Try to build a rapport through the tone of your voice.

Data gathering
- A detailed history is essential in the absence of physical examination and signs.
- Use open and focused/closed questions to include/exclude relevant conditions.

Summarising
- Ensure that you have established the patient's ideas, concerns and expectations.
- Allow time for the patient to ask questions.

Clinical management

- Agree on a plan of action and give clear information about when to seek further advice or help (safety net).
- Request that the patient repeats the advice given.
- Allow the patient to end the call first.

Documentation

- Accurate records should be kept for all telephone consultations, with details of the management plan and follow-up agreed with the patient.

Role play

Information for doctor	Additional information for role player
Patient: Master JA *Age:* 8 months *PMH:* Nil *DH:* Nil *Information:* Mrs A (JA's mother) contacted the surgery this morning for telephone advice as JA has had a fever. You are a locum GP.	*PC:* Fever since last night (39°C). Diarrhoea 6x since last night. Vomited 5x. *HPC:* JA has not been eating or drinking much. Has been giving him regular Calpol. **Only 1 wet nappy today. Lethargic. Not as active. No rash.** *ICE:* **Mum worried as he is not keeping fluids down. Has been trying bottles of milk so far.** Would like him to be seen at the surgery.

Home visit

- Home visits still remain an integral part of primary care, although their use is diminishing.
- In 1995, 9% of all GP consultations in the UK were home visits, whereas in 2006 this had decreased to just 4% (ONS and DoH Survey).
- GPs tend to visit a patient at home when the patient is confined due to illness or disability, or when urgent treatment can be given more quickly by visiting.
- The disadvantage of a home visit is that it is very time consuming for the GP and there is not access to some medical equipment which might otherwise be available in the surgery.

Framework for home visit consultations

Preparation

- Ensure you read through the patient's notes prior to visiting, familiarizing yourself with the patient's past medical history, medication history, allergies and recent consultations. It is useful to take a print out of this information on a home visit.
- Ensure that you pack a doctors' bag with all the relevant equipment.

- Ring the patient beforehand to determine the reason for the home visit request and confirm with them that you will be visiting.
- To ensure your safety, let a member of staff know that you are going on a home visit and give the details of which patient you are visiting.

Data gathering

- Ask open questions, followed by focused questions including those to check for red flags.
- Establish social history: Is the patient coping at home? Is additional help required?
- Examination .

Clinical management

- Decide if the patient is safe to remain at home or if they need to be referred to hospital.
- Are any further investigations required?
- Is any medication required?
- Safety net.
- Clearly document the consultation when back at the surgery.

Role play

Information for doctor	Additional information for role player
Patient: Mrs JL *Age*: 90 years *SH*: Lives alone in a 1 bedroom ground floor flat. Has carers twice daily. *PMH*: COPD *DH*: Tiotropium 18 mcg 2 puffs daily; Seretide 250 mcg 1 puff twice daily *Information*: Patient's daughter phoned this morning requesting a visit for her mother as she has been increasingly breathless. You are a GP Registrar.	*PC*: *"I've had a bit of a cough over the past few days and can't walk very far without getting very breathless".* *PMH*: **Cough productive of green sputum.** Haven't been able to get out of the house. **No chest pain. No fever.** *SH*: **Ex-smoker (gave up 15 yrs ago).** *ICE*: *"I think my COPD is getting worse".* *O/E*: Coarse crackles on right side of chest. Apyrexial.

Angry patient

- Managing an angry patient can be upsetting and potentially dangerous.
- The reason for a patient being angry can include anything from social or financial problems to difficulties getting GP appointments, poor communication, or a doctor ignoring their ideas, concerns and expectations.
- An angry patient can escalate to a violent patient. Signs of escalation include shouting, swearing, raising a clenched fist, pacing or adopting an aggressive posture.

Tips for managing an angry patient

- Remain calm.
- Start with an open question – *"Can you tell me about what's upsetting you?".*
- Give the patient space and time to vent their anger.
- Apologise, for example by saying *"I'm sorry you've had to go through this".*
- Do not blame others, for example, colleagues.
- Be empathic and express concern where appropriate.
- Listen to the patient and explore their concerns.
- Agree an appropriate management plan, for example, raising the issue at the next practice meeting.
- Offer details of how the patient can make a formal complaint. A complaint to the practice manager will usually be acknowledged within two working days and responded to within ten working days, although this varies between practices.
- Housekeeping – it is also important to look after your own well-being.

Role play

Information for doctor	Additional information for role player
Patient: Mrs TT *Age*: 32 years *SH*: Lives with partner, unemployed, no children *PMH*: NIDDM *DH*: Metformin 850 mg BD *Information*: You are a salaried GP.	*PC*: *"I've had a sore throat for over a week and I'm very angry because I've been trying to see a doctor for days and I have never been able to get an appointment".* *HPC*: Not happy with the appointment system. **No fever. No earache. No cough.** *ICE*: **Wants antibiotics to get rid of the sore throat.** Will get angry if she doesn't get these unless a suitable explanation is given. *O/E*: Apyrexial; normal ENT and chest examination.

Breaking bad news

- Breaking bad news is a duty which understandably many GPs dread, but is nevertheless a necessary skill to learn well.

Tips for breaking bad news

Preparation

- Arrange a face to face meeting and not a telephone consultation.
- Ensure no interruptions.
- Invite a relative or friend if appropriate.
- Prepare beforehand by familiarising yourself with the patient's clinical details.

Data gathering

- Discover what information the patient already knows or what they have been told so far.
- Discover what has happened since the patient was last seen.
- Give the patient a warning shot that difficult information is to follow, for example: "*I'm afraid that it looks more serious than we had hoped*" or "*I'm afraid that it is rather bad news*".
- Share the information in small 'chunks', clearly and honestly, repeating the salient points. Allow pauses where appropriate.
- Avoid jargon.
- Continue to check the patient's understanding.
- Be aware of the patient's non-verbal cues as this can help to gauge the patient's need for further information.
- Show empathy, for example, "*I know that this must be very difficult for you*".
- Address the patient's ideas, concerns and expectations.

Clinical management

- Decide on a management plan which should include some sort of follow-up appointment and safety net.
- Offer some hope but this should also be tempered with realism.
- Offer a patient information leaflet if appropriate.
- Identify the patient's support network.
- Offer to make another appointment with spouse/relative or to speak to them on the phone.

Role play

Information for doctor	Additional information for role player
Patient: Mrs ZS *Age*: 42 years *SH*: Married with 5 children *PMH*: Nil *DH*: Nil *Information*: Saw the salaried GP 4 weeks ago due to a breast lump. Was seen in the breast clinic 2 weeks ago and has come for her results. You are a locum GP. *Biopsy result*: Adenocarcinoma of left breast.	*PC*: "*I was asked to come to get my biopsy results from the breast clinic*". "*Is there a problem?*". *HPC*: Felt a left breast lump 4 weeks ago. Has increased in size since. **Not painful. No nipple discharge. No skin tethering.** *FH*: **No FH of breast cancer.** *ICE*: Worried it might be breast cancer.

Patient with learning disabilities

- Learning disability is defined as a 'significantly reduced ability to understand new and complex information, to learn new skills (impaired intelligence), and with a reduced ability to cope independently (impaired social functioning)'. It starts before adulthood with a lasting effect on development. Often there are associated co-morbidities, for example, epilepsy, mental illness and behavioural disorders (*DoH White Paper*, 2001, *Valuing people: a new strategy for learning disabilities for the 21st century*).
- A consultation with a patient who has learning disabilities can be challenging for both the patient and the doctor.
- The patient may feel that their health needs have been neglected, whilst the doctor may feel frustrated by the potential difficulty in gathering the relevant clinical information to formulate a management plan.
- Evidence has shown that people with learning disabilities have much greater health needs than the general population, yet they don't access primary care as often as they need to (*NHS Primary Service Framework*, 2007, *Management of health for people with learning disabilities in primary care*).
- Management of patients with learning disabilities involves a multidisciplinary team approach.

Tips for data gathering and clinical management

- The people caring for the patient, whether the patient lives with their parents, or has a carer, or lives in a residential home, are all very useful sources of information.
- Listen to the patient and give them time to express their concerns.
- When history taking, ensure that the patient understands the questions asked and avoid using any jargon.
- It is important to try building a rapport with the patient, and ideally they should see the same GP each visit.
- When giving information, writing things down can be useful if the patient is literate. Drawing diagrams or giving patient information leaflets can also be helpful.
- All patients with learning disabilities should have at least an annual health check, and should have an individualised 'health action plan' (*DoH White Paper*, 2001, *Valuing people: a new strategy for learning disabilities for the 21st century*).
- A health check should include a minimum of:
  - provision of relevant health promotion advice
  - chronic illness and system enquiry
  - physical examination
  - consideration of whether the patient suffers from epilepsy, any mental health or behavioural problems
  - specific syndrome check
  - medication review
  - review of co-ordination arrangements with other healthcare providers.

Role play

Information for doctor	Additional information for role player
Patient: Mr TB *Age*: 36 years *SH*: Lives in a residential home for people with learning disabilities. *PMH*: Down syndrome, hypothyroidism, mild hearing impairment. *DH*: Levothyroxine 75 mcg OD *Information*: Was last seen by GP 8 months ago for ear infection. You are a salaried GP.	*PC*: *"I've got tummy pains doc,' 'I've had it for a few days and it's really bad".* *HPC*: Lower abdominal pain, mainly left-sided. Intermittent pain. **Last opened bowels 5 days ago. No urinary symptoms. No D&V. No fever.** Not taken any painkillers so far. **Doesn't have much fibre in his diet.** *ICE*: Worried about his appendix. *O/E*: Apyrexial. Abdo soft. No organomegaly. Palpable mass in LIF.

Patient with hearing impairment

- Hearing impairment in general practice is a relatively common problem; however, research suggests that the needs of this patient group are poorly met in many GP surgeries (Patient UK, 2009, *Survey of people with mild to profound hearing loss*).
- The problems that patients with hearing impairment face include problems trying to book appointments, not hearing their name being called by the doctor, not being offered an interpreter, and not being able to understand the doctor.
- In the CSA exam there may be a hearing impaired patient, and they would most likely communicate by lip reading.
- When communicating with a hearing impaired patient, it is vital to ensure that you communicate clearly, with good face to face contact, and regularly check patient understanding.

Tips for dealing with hearing-impaired patients

- Always ask the patient at the beginning of the consultation how they wish to communicate.
- Always look at the patient when listening and speaking.
- Avoid looking at the patient's notes when talking to the patient – look at these before the patient enters.
- Ensure you are sitting in good light and keep your hands away from your face if the patient is lip reading.
- Speak clearly but not too slowly.
- Don't exaggerate lip movements if the patient is lip reading.
- Keep a pen and paper handy in case you need to write anything down.
- Ask the patient to summarise what has been said to ensure understanding.
- Offer additional written material at the end of the consultation.
- Drawing diagrams to explain things may be especially useful in this case.

Role play

Information for doctor	Additional information for role player
Patient: Mrs RA *Age*: 48 years *SH*: Lives with husband and 3 children. Housewife *FH*: Nil *PMH*: IBS *DH*: Nil *Information*: You are a GP Registrar.	*PC*: *"I've been having problems with my hearing for the past month or so"*. *HPC*: Can't hear on left side. **No tinnitus. No headache. No earache. No dizziness.** Never had hearing tested before. **No trauma.** *ICE*: Worried she might be going deaf. **Would like a hearing test.** *O/E*: Decreased hearing on left side. Abnormal Weber's test – sound localised to right ear.

Healthy people: promoting health and preventing disease

Hypercholesterolaemia

- Refers to a high level of lipids in the blood stream.
- It is more specifically defined as an elevation in total cholesterol, low density lipoproteins or triglycerides in the bloodstream.
- Fatty lumps called atheromas can develop in the lining of the blood vessels if the cholesterol remains high.
- A build up of atheroma can result in ischaemic heart disease, stroke, TIA or other arterial disease developing.
- Other risk factors for atheroma formation include high blood pressure, obesity, diabetes, unhealthy diet and strong family history.
- The figure below shows how you can illustrate the effect of atheromas on blood vessels.

Normal artery

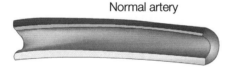

Narrowing artery

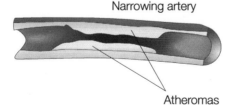

Atheromas

Data gathering

Open questions
- *"I gather you recently had a cholesterol test done. Do you mind telling me what you understand about this test?"*

- *"What do you know about having high cholesterol?"*
- *"Tell me about your diet?"*

Focused/closed questions

HPC: *"Do you have any chest pain or shortness of breath?"*

PMH: *"Do you have any history of high blood pressure, high cholesterol, heart disease or diabetes?"*

SH: Smoking/alcohol/illicit drug history? Exercise?

FH: *"Do any of your family have high cholesterol or heart disease?"*

ICE: *"Do you have any thoughts as to why your cholesterol is high?"*

Examination:
- blood pressure
- BMI
- cardiovascular system, including inspection for xanthelasma and tendon xanthomas.

Clinical management

Investigations
- Fasting cholesterol screen – total serum cholesterol, HDL, LDL, triglycerides.
- Fasting glucose.
- LFTs – if starting statins.
- U&Es – to check kidney function.

Explanation to patient
- Cholesterol is a fat made in the liver from the foods that we eat.
- A small amount of cholesterol is beneficial in keeping us healthy.
- If the cholesterol level is too high (above 5 mmol/l), there is an increased risk of developing heart problems or having a stroke.
- Cholesterol is carried in the bloodstream by particles called lipoproteins. There are two types of lipoproteins: low density lipoproteins (LDL) and high density lipoproteins (HDL). The LDL are often referred to as the 'bad' cholesterol as they are thought to be responsible for atheroma formation, whereas HDL are referred to as the 'good' cholesterol as they are thought to prevent atheroma formation.
- It is therefore important to keep the cholesterol level down to an acceptable level (≤5 mmol/l).

Management (based on *NICE* 2010 guideline CG67: *Lipid modification*)
- Use a CVD risk calculator to help explain the risk to patients (e.g. Framingham 1991 10-year risk equation).
- Cardio-protective diet – fewer saturated fats, less alcohol, at least five portions of fruit and vegetables each day, and two portions of fish per week.
- Weight management and exercise – 30 minutes of at least moderate intensity exercise at least 5 days a week.

- Smoking cessation.
- Medication: initiate statins for primary prevention of CVD if 10-year risk ≥20%, or for secondary prevention of CVD. Preferred choice is simvastatin 40 mg OD.
- Safety net – if on statins monitor LFTs within 3 months and then 12 monthly.

Role play

Information for doctor	Additional information for role player
Patient: Mrs HB *Age*: 46 years *PMH*: Hypertension *DH*: Bendrofluazide 2.5 mg OD *Weight*: 96 kg (BMI 40) *Information*: Had a recent cholesterol test: total serum cholesterol 6.8 (NR: <5.2) serum LDL 4.2 (NR: 1.5–3.0); serum HDL 1.1 (NR: >1.0) serum triglycerides 2.0 (NR: <1.7) You are a locum GP.	*PC*: *"I have come to get my cholesterol results"*. *HPC*: No symptoms. Feels well. **Doesn't drink any alcohol but cooks with a lot of oils and eats a lot of cheese.** *FH*: **Mother had high cholesterol. Father has diabetes.** *ICE*: Not keen to start a cholesterol tablet as doesn't like taking tablets. Would rather try to change her diet.

Hypertension

- Blood pressure means the pressure of the blood in your arteries (blood vessels).
- Approximately half of all people over 65 years have high blood pressure (hypertension).
- Hypertension is defined in adults as a diastolic blood pressure persistently above 90 mmHg, and/or a systolic blood pressure persistently above 140 mmHg.
- It is recommended that GPs diagnose hypertension only after obtaining two or more elevated blood pressure readings on separate occasions.
- Risk factors for hypertension include obesity, inactivity, alcohol and smoking.
- Hypertension can result in an increased risk of ischaemic heart disease and stroke.

Data gathering

Open question
- *"Your recent blood pressure check has shown that your blood pressure is higher than normal. What do you understand about high blood pressure?"*

Focused/closed questions
HPC: *"Do you have any headaches or problems with your vision? Any chest pain?"*

PMH: *"Do you have any history of high blood pressure, heart disease or stroke?"*

SH: Smoking/alcohol/illicit drug history? Diet? Exercise? Occupation? Stress?

FH: *"Does anyone else in the family have high blood pressure?"*

ICE: *"Do you have any thoughts as to why your blood pressure might be high?"*

Examination:
- re-check BP
- fundoscopy
- BMI
- cardiovascular system

Clinical management

Investigations
- Bloods – U&Es, fasting cholesterol & glucose.
- ECG.
- Urine dipstick – check for protein and blood (red flag if microscopic haematuria).

Explanation to patient
- Blood pressure measurements consist of two readings – the top reading records the highest pressure in the arteries when the heart contracts. The bottom reading records the lowest pressure in the arteries as the heart relaxes between beats.
- If either of these readings are high then you have high blood pressure (above 140/90 mmHg).
- High blood pressure can be due to genetic factors, high salt or alcohol intake, lack of exercise or stress.
- If your blood pressure remains high you are at increased risk of having a heart attack or a stroke.
- It is therefore important that your blood pressure is kept within an acceptable range and it should be monitored regularly.

Management
- Lifestyle advice – reduce salt and alcohol intake, increased exercise, smoking cessation.
- Offer anti-hypertensive medication to patients with persistent high blood pressure of 160/100 mmHg or more, or to those patients with a 10-year CVD risk above 20% and blood pressure above 140/90 mmHg (*NICE*, 2006, CG34: *Hypertension*).
- In hypertensive patients aged 55 or older, or black patients of any age, the first choice drug for initial therapy is either a calcium channel blocker or a thiazide diuretic.
- In hypertensive patients younger than 55, the first choice is an ACE inhibitor (or angiotensin-II receptor antagonist if unable to tolerate an ACE inhibitor).

- Refer immediately if any signs of malignant hypertension (BP >180/110 mmHg with papilloedema +/- retinal haemorrhage) or phaeochromocytoma (signs include headache, palpitations and excessive sweating).
- Safety net – review hypertensive patients annually or more frequently if poorly controlled blood pressure. Advise patients to see GP or go to A&E if they develop any of the symptoms above.

Role play

Information for doctor	Additional information for role player
Patient: Mr JB *Age*: 57 years *SH*: Farm labourer, smokes 10 cigs/day, alcohol intake 30 units/wk *PMH*: Gout *DH*: Allopurinol *Information*: Registered with practice last week. BP on registration 180/95 mmHg. You are a GP partner.	*PC*: "*I was asked to book an appointment to get my BP checked*". *HPC*: Feels well; no headache or visual symptoms. Doesn't understand why he needed to come back as he feels fine. **Eats a lot of takeaways. No exercise except for job.** *ICE*: No concerns. *O/E*: BP 175/98 mmHg; weight 100 kg (BMI 34); CVS exam NAD.

Obesity

- Often classified as a BMI of over 30.
- BMI is defined as an individual's body weight (in kilograms) divided by the square of his or her height (in metres). It provides a good estimate as to whether an individual is in a healthy weight range by taking into consideration their height.
- Approximately 1 in 5 adults in the UK are obese. (*NHS Information Centre, 2010, Statistics on obesity, physical activity and diet*).

Data gathering

Open question
- "*Your current weight places you in the obese range... can you tell me a bit more about your lifestyle in terms of diet and exercise?*".

Focused/closed questions
HPC: "*How much exercise do you do in an average week?*"
"*Does your diet contain a lot of fatty &/or sugary foods?*"
"*Have you previously tried to lose weight?*"
"*Any breathlessness or chest pain?*" (red flags)
"*Any tiredness or problems sleeping?*"
"*Any bowel symptoms?*"
PMH: Any history of high blood pressure, high cholesterol or diabetes?

SH: Smoking history? Alcohol? Occupation?

FH: *"Do any of your family have weight problems?"*

ICE: *"Do you have any particular concerns about your weight?"*
"What were you hoping we could do to help you?"

Examination:
- BMI (>25 overweight; >30 obese; >40 morbidly obese)
- BP
- cardiovascular system – to check for secondary problems

Clinical management

Investigations
- Blood test – fasting cholesterol/glucose, U&Es, LFTs, TSH. LH/FSH in females if excluding PCOS.

Explanation to patient
- Obesity is defined as a BMI of over 30.
- The BMI provides a good estimate of how much of your body is made up of fat.
- When you are overweight or obese, it simply means that your energy intake exceeds energy expenditure.
- If you are overweight or obese you are at increased risk of developing health problems such as diabetes, high blood pressure, heart disease, or some types of cancer.

Management
- Low calorie/low fat diet (more fruit and vegetables, fish and lean meats, fewer sugary drinks, grilling instead of frying, etc.).
- Increase exercise.
- Decrease alcohol intake.
- Anti-obesity medications – Orlistat 120 mg TDS:
  - interferes with the way that fats are digested and absorbed in the body.
  - can only be prescribed for patients with a BMI of >30 or >28 with an associated health problem (*NICE*, 2010, *CG43: Obesity*).
  - side effects include fatty stools, excess wind and increased urgency.
  - patients must lose at least 5% of their body weight in the first 3 months to continue with this medication (*NICE*, 2010, *CG43: Obesity*).
- Surgery, e.g. gastric band/gastric bypass (NICE criteria for bariatric surgery includes BMI >40 or >35 with other co-morbidities and when other treatments have failed (*NICE*, 2006, *CG43: Obesity*).

Role play

Information for doctor	Additional information for role player
Patient: Mrs JN *Age*: 37 years *SH*: Married, works as chef. Non-smoker; 5 units alcohol/wk. *PMH*: NIDDM *DH*: Metformin 850 mg TDS *Information*: Had review with nurse last week: Weight 98 kg, BMI 38. You are a locum GP.	*PC*: "*I would like some of those weight loss tablets doctor*." *HPC*: Has been trying to lose weight for months. Feels that she eats healthily but still doesn't lose any weight. **Doesn't have time for exercise. Snacks at work. Typically skips breakfast. Eats chicken mayonnaise sandwich for lunch and often curry with rice for dinner.** *FH*: Nil. *ICE*: Would like some weight loss tablets. *O/E*: Weight 99 kg; BP 140/86 mmHg; CVS exam – NAD.

Smoking cessation

- Cigarette smoking is the single greatest cause of illness and premature death in the UK.
- Approximately 100 000 people die each year in the UK as a result of smoking-related illnesses.
- Stopping smoking can be very beneficial to a person's health and well-being.

Data gathering

Open question
- "*So tell me a bit more about why you have decided to give up smoking?*" "*Why now?*"

Focused/closed questions
HPC: "*How many cigarettes are you currently smoking a day?*"
"*When did you first start smoking?*"
"*Have you ever tried to give up smoking before?*"
"*When is your predicted stop date?*"
"*Any breathlessness, coughing up blood or weight loss?*" (red flags)
PMH: Any medical conditions?
DH: Do you take any regular medications? (bupropion taken with certain medications, e.g. anti-psychotics or anti-depressants, increases the risk of seizures)
FH: "*Is there any history of cancer, lung disease or heart disease in the family?*"
SH: Alcohol/illicit drug history? Who lives with you at home? Support? Occupation?
ICE: "*What help were you hoping for in terms of stopping smoking?*"

Examination: Nothing specific although if there are signs of chest symptoms do a respiratory examination.

Clinical management

Investigations
- Nothing specific although if there are any chest symptoms consider spirometry or CXR.

Explanation to patient
- Nicotine is a drug that is inhaled from the tobacco in cigarettes.
- Nicotine is the addictive ingredient in cigarettes – as the blood level of nicotine falls, people develop withdrawal symptoms, for example, anxiety, irritability, headaches and difficulty concentrating.
- By replacing the nicotine or mimicking the effects of the nicotine, there are substitution treatments that can help when trying to stop smoking.

Management
- Patient information leaflet – www.patient.co.uk - *'Tips to help you stop smoking'.*
- Local NHS smoking cessation service or support groups.
- Nicotine replacement therapy – stops or reduces the symptoms of nicotine withdrawal (available in gum, patches, lozenges, etc.).
- Varenicline (Champix) – mimics the effects of nicotine on the body. Standard treatment course is 12 weeks. Side effects include nausea, insomnia, abnormal dreams and less commonly mood changes. Should not be used if under 18, pregnant, breast-feeding or if severe renal disease. Use with caution in patients with a history of psychiatric illness.
- Buproprion (Zyban) – alters the level of some chemicals in the brain that seem to relieve the withdrawal symptoms associated with stopping smoking. Standard treatment course is 8 weeks. Side effects include dry mouth, insomnia and, rarely, seizures. It should not be used if under 18, pregnant, breast-feeding or if the patient has ever had epilepsy or a seizure. Also not advisable in certain psychiatric conditions. See BNF for further details.
- Offer regular follow-up and support.

Role play

Information for doctor	Additional information for role player
Patient: Mrs JS *Age*: 42 years *SH*: Receptionist, married, lives with husband and 2 children. *PMH*: Myocardial infarction 2009 *DH*: Aspirin 75 mg OD; simvastatin 40 mg OD. *Information*: You are a GP Registrar	*PC*: *"I would like to give up smoking".* *HPC*: Has smoked 20 cigs/day for past 25 years. Has not tried to quit before. Her children have been nagging her to quit. No shortness of breath and no weight loss. *SH*: Alcohol 12 units/wk *ICE*: **Keen to quit smoking as had a heart attack last year which scared her.**

Genetics in primary care

Antenatal screening for Down syndrome

- Down syndrome is a chromosomal abnormality in which there is an extra copy of chromosome number 21 (often known as trisomy 21).
- Characteristic features of Down syndrome include macroglossia, epicanthic folds, upslanting palpebral fissures and a single transverse palmar crease. Individuals with Down syndrome have a higher incidence of congenital heart defects, gastro-oesophageal reflux, recurrent ear infections and thyroid problems.
- Down syndrome can be diagnosed either before birth (antenatally) or after birth.
- The latest NICE guidelines recommend that all pregnant women should be offered screening for Down syndrome.
- There are two different types of tests that can be done in pregnancy – a screening test and a diagnostic test.
  - Screening test – looks at the chance of a baby being born with Down syndrome in the current pregnancy.
  - Diagnostic test – amniocentesis or chorionic villus sampling is used to give a definite diagnosis as to whether or not the fetus has Down syndrome. Usually only done if the screening test indicates a high chance of Down syndrome (usually >1/250 risk).
- Screening tests used include:
  - The combined test is the one which NICE currently recommends. This includes a nuchal translucency scan (measures the size of the nuchal pad at the nape of the fetal neck) and blood tests for serum PAPP-A and β-hCG (undertaken between 11 weeks and 13 weeks^{+6}).
  - Amniocentesis – a sample of amniotic fluid is taken from the amniotic sac using a fine needle. This is normally done at 15 weeks of gestation and carries an additional 1% risk of miscarriage.
  - CVS – a small sample of tissue is taken from part of the placenta called the chorionic villi. Normally done at 11^{+0}–13^{+6} weeks of gestation (*RCOG*, 2010: *Green-top guideline 8: Amniocentesis and chorionic villus sampling*) and carries an approximately 2% risk of miscarriage.

Data gathering

Open question

- *"What do you know about Down syndrome and the antenatal screening tests available?"*.

Focused/closed questions

HPC: *"Is this your first pregnancy?"*
If not, any problems in previous pregnancies? Miscarriages? TOP?
"Have you had Down screening in previous pregnancies? Any concerns?"

SH: "Who lives with you at home?" Occupation? Support?

FH: Does anyone in the family have Down syndrome?

ICE: *"Do you have concerns about the risk of Down syndrome?"*
"Do you know anyone with Down syndrome?"

Examination:
- BP
- Routine antenatal examination

Clinical management

Investigations

- Screening tests (see www.patient.co.uk article *'Antenatal Screening for Down's Syndrome'* for further details).
- Amniocentesis.
- CVS.

Explanation to patient

- Down syndrome is a genetic disorder where a person inherits an extra copy of one chromosome. The additional genetic material changes the finely tuned balance of the body, resulting in characteristic physical features and affects the normal physical development.

Management

- Give patient information leaflet.
- Follow up after the screening/diagnostic tests.
- Refer to obstetrician and geneticist if Down syndrome confirmed antenatally.

Role play

Information for doctor	Additional information for role player
Patient: Mrs TW *Age*: 40 years *PMH*: Hypothyroidism *DH*: Levothyroxine 100 mcg daily *SH*: Lives with husband, works as a solicitor, currently 8 weeks pregnant (1st pregnancy) *Information*: You are a salaried GP.	PC: Would like referral for antenatal Down syndrome screening and would like to know more about what the screening entails. HPC: Has heard about amniocentesis but was told there were some other tests available. ICE: **Worried about the risk of Down syndrome due to her age. Her sister has a child with Down syndrome.**

Screening for sickle cell disease

- Antenatal screening is available for sickle cell conditions in certain parts of the UK.
- Sickle cell disease is most common in people of African–Caribbean descent.
- For a baby to be affected with sickle cell disease both parents must have the sickle cell gene. Sickle cell disease causes chronic haemolytic anaemia, dactylitis, painful acute crises and increases the risk of stroke, organ damage and bacterial infections. Average life expectancy is about 50 years.
- Sickle cell trait occurs in people with one sickle cell gene and one normal gene. People with sickle cell trait do not usually have any clinical manifestation of illness.
- Pregnant women and couples planning to conceive may want to know whether they have sickle cell trait, because if they both have the gene their child might inherit sickle cell disease.

Data gathering

Open question
- *"What do you know about sickle cell conditions and the antenatal screening available?"*

Focused/closed questions
HPC: *"Is this your first pregnancy?"*
If not, any previous problems, for example miscarriages, TOP?
"Have you or your partner ever been screened for sickle cell trait before?"
"Have you or your partner ever had problems with recurrent infections or lethargy before?"

FH: *"Do you know of any family history of sickle cell disease or trait?"*

DH Do you take any regular medications?

SH: Smoking/alcohol/illicit drug history? Who lives with you at home? Support? Occupation?

ICE: *"Do you have any worries/concerns about sickle cell screening?"*
"Do you know anyone with sickle cell disease?"

Clinical management

Investigations
- Blood test called haemoglobin electrophoresis (offer to father also if mother carries the sickle cell gene).
- FBC – check Hb.

Explanation to patient
- Sickle cell disease is an inherited blood disorder which causes the red cells in the bloodstream to become sickle-shaped.

- When sickle-shaped cells block small blood vessels, less blood can reach that part of the body. This can result in damage to those affected tissues. This is what causes the complications of sickle cell disease.

Management
- Pre- and post-test counselling.
- Give information leaflet on sickle cell screening (http://sct.screening.nhs.uk/index.php).
- Refer to obstetrician and haematologist if both parents are carriers of the sickle cell gene.

Role play

Information for doctor	Additional information for role player
Patient: Ms CC *Age*: 28 years *SH*: Retail assistant. *DH*: Nil *Information*: Saw locum GP 1 week ago for antenatal booking – 6 weeks pregnant.	*PC*: *"I would like to get screened for the sickle cell gene as my partner has sickle cell trait and I'm currently pregnant."* *HPC*: Never been screened before. **Doesn't know much about sickle cell disease.** No symptoms. *ICE*: Would like to find out more about screening and sickle cell disease. First pregnancy.

Cystic fibrosis

- Autosomal recessive condition mainly affecting the lungs, pancreas and digestive system.
- Symptoms begin in early childhood and include recurrent chest infections, malabsorption of food and failure to thrive.
- Treatment includes antibiotics, pancreatic enzyme replacements, chest physiotherapy and mucolytics.
- Approximately 1 in 25 people of Caucasian descent are carriers of the cystic fibrosis gene in the UK.

Data gathering

Open question
- *"Please can you tell me a bit more about your concerns?"*

Focused/closed questions
HPC: *"Have you been pregnant before? If so, any miscarriages or termination of pregnancies?"*
"Have you had any problems with antenatal scans before?"

"Have you or your partner been tested for the CF gene before?"
"Do you have children with any symptoms such as poor weight gain or recurrent chest infections?"
FH: *"Does anyone in the family have cystic fibrosis?"*
ICE: *"What concerns do you have about the possibility of having cystic fibrosis?"*
"Do you know anyone with cystic fibrosis?"
Examination: Routine antenatal examination (if patient is pregnant)
N.B. No children are used in the CSA examination so you will not be expected to examine a child.

Clinical management

Investigations

- Genetic testing prenatally – blood test or scrapings from the inside of the mouth can be used to check for the cystic fibrosis gene in the parents.
- Antenatal testing – uses chorionic villus sampling and is carried out from 10 weeks of pregnancy.
- After birth, a sweat test can be used to diagnose cystic fibrosis and blood from the Guthrie heel prick test is routinely screened for cystic fibrosis by checking for increased levels of immuno-reactive trypsinogen (IRT) at around 7 days of age.

Explanation to patient

- In order to get cystic fibrosis you have to inherit two cystic fibrosis genes, one from your mother and one from your father.
- In cystic fibrosis, a pair of genes on chromosome 7 don't work properly.
- These genes are responsible for the way cells handle salt and water and they control mucus secretions. When you have cystic fibrosis water and salt aren't transported out of cells so efficiently and as a result, the mucus secretions are thicker than normal; these sticky secretions are difficult to clear from the body leading to increased lung infections and damage to the digestive system.

Management

- If one or both parents carry the cystic fibrosis gene, refer for genetic counselling.
- Provide a patient information leaflet.

Role play

Information for doctor	Additional information for role player
Patient: Mrs JT *Age*: 31 years *SH*: Married, has 1 child with cystic fibrosis *PMH*: Asthma *DH*: Salbutamol, beclomethasone. *Information*: You are a GP Partner.	*PC*: Currently pregnant and worried about the risk of cystic fibrosis. *HPC*: Would like to get checked for whether the 2nd child will have cystic fibrosis. 8 weeks pregnant. *ICE*: Very worried about the 2nd child also having CF. Wants further screening.

Care of acutely ill people

Suicidal patient

- Suicide can be described as a fatal act of self harm, initiated with the intention of ending one's own life.
- Self harm describes the deliberate act of harming oneself.
- All health professionals should be vigilant of patients who express a desire to harm themselves, and these patients should have a suicide risk assessment undertaken.
- Risk factors for suicide include male gender, elderly, unemployed, history of mental illness or past suicide attempt, alcohol or drug abuse and poor social support.

Data gathering

Open question
- *"Please can you tell me how you are currently feeling, and what has triggered these suicidal thoughts?"*

Focused/closed questions

HPC: *"How is your sleep/your concentration/your energy levels/your mood/your self-esteem?"*
"Have you made specific plans for suicide? If so, what are these plans?"
See suicide risk assessment below for further questions.

PMH: Any past history of psychiatric illness? Any previous history of suicide/self harm?

DH: *"Are you on any regular medications such as anti-depressants?"*

SH: *"Is there anyone with you at home who can offer you support?"*
Smoking history/alcohol/illicit drug use? Occupation?

FH: Any FH of suicide/mental illness?

Examination: Mental state examination (see *Appendix 3*).

Clinical management

Investigations
- Suicide risk assessment
  - *"Do you have any plan to harm yourself or others?"* (red flag)
  - *"Have you been thinking about this for a while or are these just fleeting thoughts?"*
  - *"How do you plan to end your life?"*

- "How seriously do you intend on acting on these thoughts?" (red flag)
- "What would stop you?"
- "Any previous suicide attempts or self harming episodes – how many?" (red flag)
- "Any history of substance abuse?"
- "Have you ever been in trouble with the police before?" "Have you ever been in prison before?"
- "Any current contributing life stressors (financial, relationships, family, etc)?"
- "Any symptoms of depression or psychosis?"
- "Do you have any hope for the future?"
- "Do you have any chronic medical conditions/terminal illness that may be contributing?"
- "Do you feel isolated, lonely, angry or impulsive?"
- "How do you cope with these issues?" "Do you feel able to talk to anyone about your problems?"

Management

- If low suicide risk, offer regular follow-up and consider referral to the local mental health services.
- If moderate–high suicide risk refer urgently to the mental health crisis team.
- Give contact details of the Samaritans or the local crisis team if appropriate.
- Always safety net – inform them of how they can access help if things get worse.

Role play

Information for doctor	Additional information for role player
Patient: Mr JS *Age*: 23 years *SH*: Lives alone, unemployed. *PMH*: Depression, previous psychiatric admission due to severe depression 2009. No forensic history. *DH*: Mirtazepine 60 mg *Information*: You are a locum GP.	*PC*: "I can't carry on like this" "I don't feel like living any more". *HPC*: No specific plans for suicide. Feels hopeless as no job and struggling to pay bills. Low mood: **Doesn't feel able to talk to family. Waking up several times in the night.** No previous suicide or self harm attempts. Feels little hope for the future. *ICE*: **Would like some urgent help as feels suicidal.**

Chest pain

- Can be divided into cardiac, respiratory, musculoskeletal or gastrointestinal causes.
- It is important to exclude a life threatening cause of chest pain, such as a myocardial infarction or a pulmonary embolism.

Data gathering

Open question

- *"Please can you describe the chest pain that you've been having?"*

Focused/closed questions

HPC: *"Where is the site of the chest pain? Does the pain spread anywhere else?"*
"What type of pain is it?"
"Is the pain intermittent or constant?"
"How severe is the pain out of 10?"
"Does anything make the pain better/worse?"
"Have you coughed up any blood or noticed any calf pain?" (red flags)
Any SOB, palpitations, cough or vomiting?
Any sweating or clamminess? (red flag)

PMH: Any previous heart attack or angina? Any previous surgery?

DH: *"Are you on any regular medications?"*

SH: Smoking/alcohol/illicit drug history? Occupation?

ICE: *"Do you have any idea what might be causing this chest pain?"*
"Are you concerned about anything in particular?"
"How has this pain been affecting you?"

Examination:
- BP
- Cardiac and respiratory examination
- Examine chest wall for any tenderness
- Examine calves for any swelling (DVT)
- Abdominal examination if indicated from the history

Clinical management

Investigations

- Routine bloods – FBC, U&Es, LFTs, TFTs, fasting glucose and lipids
- ECG
- CXR – if indicated

Management

- Depends on the diagnosis:
  - For non-acute chest pain consider referral to the rapid access chest pain clinic
  - If acute chest pain or any suggestion of a pulmonary embolus, refer urgently to A&E by ambulance
- Safety net – if pain not improving or if worsening to return to GP or go straight to A&E.

Role play

Information for doctor	Additional information for role player
Patient: Mr JC *Age*: 53 years *SH*: Lives with wife and 2 children. Estate agent. *PMH*: Hypertension *DH*: Coracten XL 30 mg daily *Information*: Saw nurse 1 week ago for BP check (150/89 mmHg). You are a GP Registrar.	*PC*: Chest pain. *HPC*: Pain in centre of chest which started yesterday. Pain on exertion only. Slight SOB. No palpitations or cough. No fever and no sweating. No calf pain. *FH*: Father had MI aged 60 years. *ICE*: Worried about his heart. Hoping for a scan to check his heart. *O/E*: Cardiac and respiratory examination – NAD. No chest wall tenderness.

Meningitis

- Inflammation of the lining of the brain and spinal cord (meninges)
- Most commonly caused by a bacterial or viral infection
- If bacteria multiply and release toxins into the blood, it can cause septicaemia which is life threatening

Data gathering

Open question
- *"What concerns do you have about your child?"*

Focused/closed questions

HPC: *"Have you noticed a rash on your child?"*

"Any fever, neck stiffness, headache, vomiting or sensitivity to light?" (red flags)

"Has your child been more drowsy or floppy than usual?" (red flags)

"Has your child been more irritable or crying more than usual?"

"Has your child been feeding OK?"

"Has your child had any episodes of fitting?" (red flags)

"Have you noticed any changes with his/her breathing?"

"Has your child been passing urine as usual?" (red flag if decreased urine output)

"Do you have any concerns about your child's growth and development?"

PMH: Any previous history of infections or illnesses?

SH: Where are you currently living? University/school accommodation?

FH: Any family history of any illnesses?

ICE: *"What do you think might be causing his/her symptoms?"*

Examination:
- No child examination in the CSA, but there may be a telephone consultation.
- Parents can check temperature and do the 'glass test' if at home.

Clinical management

Investigations
- Blood test – FBC, U&Es, coagulation profile, blood glucose, blood culture.
- Urine MC&S and virology.
- CSF culture and serology.

Explanation to patient
- Meningitis is a swelling of the tissues around the brain and is usually caused by an infection.
- The symptoms often develop quickly and urgent treatment is needed with antibiotic injections. An antibiotic injection would be given immediately by the GP if suspected bacterial meningitis or meningococcal septicaemia. The patient would also be transferred to secondary care as an emergency by dialling 999.
- If meningitis is suspected, a sample of fluid will be taken from around the spinal cord to determine the cause.

Management
- Prevention – children are now routinely immunised against meningococcal group C and also *Haemophilus influenza* B.
- If bacterial meningitis is suspected in the community, give IM benzylpenicillin (300 mg if under 1 yr, 600 mg if 1–9 years, 1200 mg if 10 years plus) and then urgently transfer to hospital. Give prophylaxis to close contacts. Meningitis is a notifiable disease.
- Safety net – if there is a low risk of meningococcal disease the patient can be observed at home, but should be advised to go straight to A&E if they become more unwell or develop any signs of meningitis. Also arrange to review the following day in the GP surgery.

Role play

Information for doctor	Additional information for role player
Patient: Mr TD *Age:* 18 years *SH:* College student, non-smoker *PMH:* Nil *DH:* Nil *Information:* Called the practice this morning for an emergency appointment due to headache and fever. You are a salaried GP.	*PC:* Woke up this morning with fever, severe headache and rash. *HPC:* Generalised headache, photophobia and rash on his trunk. *ICE:* **Mum worried about meningitis as someone in his college recently had this, and TD didn't have his meningitis immunisation.** *O/E:* Temp. 38.9°C, photophobia, neck stiffness, petechial non-blanching rash on the chest.

Child health

Nocturnal enuresis

- Nocturnal enuresis is bed-wetting at night in a child aged 5 years or older, in the absence of congenital or acquired defects of the central nervous system or urinary tract.
- Approximately 1 in 7 children aged five, and 1 in 20 children aged ten, wet the bed.
- Primary nocturnal enuresis refers to a child who has never been dry at night, whereas secondary nocturnal enuresis implies that the child had bladder control for a period of 6 months or more before the bed-wetting started.

Data gathering

Open question
- *"Please can you tell me more about your child's bed-wetting?"*

Focused/closed questions

HPC: *"When did the bed-wetting first start?"*
"Has he/she ever been dry at night?"
"How often is it occurring?"
"Is he/she also ever wet in the day?"
"Are there any problems with his/her bowels?"
"Any other medical problems?"
"Does he/she drink many fizzy or caffeinated drinks?"
"Has he/she been passing more urine than normal or had increased thirst?" (red flags)
"Any weight loss?" (red flag)

PMH: Any other medical problems?

DH: *"Does your child take any medication?"*

SH: Any problems at home or at school? Bullying?

FH: Any family history of bed-wetting?

ICE: *"Do you have any idea as to what is causing the bed-wetting?"*
"What were you hoping we could do to help?"

Examination: • No specific examination

Clinical management

Investigations

- Urine dipstick – to check for glucose and leucocytes (not routinely recommended, however)

Explanation to parent/patient

- Urine is stored in the bladder, which stretches like a balloon as it fills up. When it stretches to a certain point, the nerves in the bladder wall send a message to the brain saying that it needs to be emptied. Urine then passes out through the urethra. If a child is asleep and the brain does not 'hear' this message, the bladder empties anyway.
- There can be many different reasons for bed-wetting including infection, constipation, too many fizzy drinks or it can be due to psychological factors.

Management (based on NICE, 2010, CG111: Nocturnal enuresis)

- Patience and reassurance.
- Do not restrict drinks but avoid caffeinated drinks before bedtime.
- Make sure your child goes to the toilet before bed, and also leave a bathroom light on so there is no fear about getting up at night.
- Treat constipation if present.
- Use a waterproof mattress cover.
- Reward system, e.g. a star chart which can be used if the child achieves a set goal.
- Bed-wetting alarm – 'conditions' children to wake and go to the toilet when their bladder is full. First line treatment if bed-wetting has not responded to the above measures.
- Desmopressin – reduces the amount of urine made at night by the kidneys. Offered to those over 7 years if rapid onset of bed-wetting and/or if short term improvement in bed-wetting is the priority of treatment.
- Safety net – if problem not improving advise to return to GP.

Role play

Information for doctor	Additional information for role player
Patient: Master JH *Age*: 8 years *PMH*: Nocturnal enuresis *DH*: Nil *Information*: Last consultation 3 months ago with salaried GP – nocturnal enuresis. Advised to try lifestyle changes and reward system. You are a locum GP.	*PC*: Mum came in today as JH's bed-wetting is no better. *HPC*: **No daytime wetting**. No other symptoms. Wet at night 3–4 times weekly. Has had periods of being dry in the past, but for the past 2 years has been bed-wetting. *SH*: Doesn't like school very much. Gets bullied. *ICE*: Would like referral to specialist as he has had this problem for 2 years and it is not getting any better.

Childhood constipation

- Describes either difficulty or straining when passing stools, passing stools less frequently than normal, or pain when passing stools.
- Causes include poor diet, inadequate fluid intake, holding stools in, or medical causes such as bowel disorders.

Data gathering

Open question

- *"Can you tell me more about the problems your child has been having with their bowels?"*

Focused/closed questions

HPC: *"When did the problem first start?"*
"How often does your child open his/her bowels?"
Any straining or pain when opening bowels?
Any blood in the stools? (red flag)
Any soiling?
Any abdominal pain?
"Are there any problems with your child's growth or development?" (red flag)

PMH: Any history of bowel problems?

SH: Any problems at home or at school?

DH: Is he/she on any regular medications?

ICE: *"Do you have any thoughts as to what is causing the constipation?"*

Examination:
- Weight and height (plot on growth chart)
- Abdominal examination
- Inspection of skin and anatomical structures of the lumbo-sacral and gluteal region.

Clinical management

Investigations

- Nothing specific.
- TFTs or coeliac antibodies if considering organic cause for constipation.
- Other investigations should only be requested by a specialist.

Explanation to parent

- Constipation is a common problem in childhood.
- It can develop for a number of reasons and does not normally indicate anything physically wrong with your child.
- Treatment can sometimes take months but symptoms do usually improve.

Management

- Dietary advice – high fibre diet, increased fluid intake, fewer fizzy drinks.
- Behavioural interventions – scheduled toileting, reward system.
- Laxatives (e.g. Movicol).
- Patient information: www.childhoodconstipation.com.
- Refer to paediatrics if no response to initial treatment within 3 months (*NICE*, 2010, *CG99: Constipation in children and young people*).

Role play

Information for doctor	Additional information for role player
Patient: Master RB *Age*: 6 years *FH*: Nil *PMH*: Nil *DH*: Nil *Information*: Mum has booked an appointment today to discuss her son RB. You are a locum GP.	*PC*: *"My son hasn't opened his bowels for 6 days"* *HPC*: Recently hard stools. No blood in stools. No abdominal pain. No other symptoms. No concerns about growth and development. **Doesn't drink much water – prefers fizzy drinks. Doesn't like fruit. Prefers crisps. Always leaves his vegetables.** *ICE*: Would like medication for his constipation. *O/E*: 75th centile for height and weight. Abdo. exam – NAD.

Attention deficit hyperactivity disorder

- ADHD is a condition affecting behaviour, which usually first presents in childhood, but can also occur in adults.
- Characterised by hyperactivity, impulsiveness and/or inattention.
- Symptoms must be present for at least 6 months, and impairment in social, academic or occupational functioning must be evident in more than one setting.
- Cause is not fully known, although it could be genetic, environmental or related to an antenatal or obstetric problem.
- Management includes multidisciplinary team involvement, methylphenidate or psychological therapy.

Data gathering

Open question

- *"Can you tell me more about your child's behaviour?"*

Focused/closed questions

HPC: *"How long have you had concerns about your child's behaviour?"*
"Is he/she more restless than most other children?"

"Have there been any concerns about him/her at school? How is he/she doing academically?"
"Have you had concerns about his/her concentration/attention at home?"
"Do you have any concerns with his/her development?"

FH: Any FH of ADHD?

DH Does your child take any regular medications?

SH Does he/she have brothers or sisters at home? How is the interaction at home with his/her siblings?

ICE: *"Do you have any thoughts as to what might be causing the behavioural problems?"*
"How is this behaviour affecting the family?"

Examination: • Height and weight (plot on growth chart)
• BP

Clinical management

Investigations

- Nothing specific.

Explanation to parent / patient

- ADHD is a common condition affecting behaviour.
- There is no simple test to diagnose ADHD.
- If your child has symptoms suggestive of ADHD, it is likely that they will be referred to a specialist who will be able to confirm the diagnosis by doing an assessment, and start any treatment if necessary.

Management

- Consider watchful waiting in mild cases. Can offer referral to parent-training/education programme or for cognitive behavioural therapy.
- If behavioural problems persist refer to secondary care.
- Medication – methylphenidate, atomoxetine or dexamfetamine (N.B. do not diagnose or start drug treatment in primary care).

Role play

Information for doctor	Additional information for role player
Patient: Master TA *Age*: 7 years *FH*: Has 2 brothers aged 9 and 10 years. Eldest brother has ADHD. *PMH*: Nil *DH*: Nil *Information*: You are a salaried GP.	*PC*: Hyperactive child, poor attention span. Teacher at school concerned as he is disruptive in class. *HPC*: **Poor concentration. Not doing well at school. Also very difficult to manage at home due to hyperactivity.** *ICE*: **Mum worried that he may have ADHD as he has very similar symptoms to his eldest brother.**

Care of older adults

Dementia

- Neurological condition causing a gradual loss of mental ability.
- It can also cause changes in personality, decline in social function and a decline in the ability to look after oneself.
- The most common cause of dementia is Alzheimer's disease, although other types include vascular dementia and Lewy body dementia.
- About 1 in 5 people over the age of 80 have dementia.
- There is no cure, although some medications can help to slow the decline in symptoms.

Data gathering

Open question
- *"What can you tell me about the memory problems you have been experiencing?"*

Focused/closed questions

HPC: *"When did you first start to notice problems with your memory?"*
"Were these changes very sudden?" (red flag)
"Is there anything in particular that you forget, for example, names, places, dates?"
"Do you have difficulty with your short term memory, long term memory or both?"
"What is your concentration like?"
"Has anyone noticed any change in your personality or mood?"
"Did you have a fall or head injury?" (red flag)

PMH: Any relevant medical conditions? Any previous operations?

DH: *"Do you take any regular medications?"*

FH: Any family history of dementia or memory problems?

SH: Who lives with you at home? Support? Any carers? Smoking/alcohol/illicit drug history?

ICE: *"What concerns do you have with your memory?"*
"How has this problem been impacting on your daily life?"

Examination:
- Neurological examination.
- Cognitive and abbreviated mental state examination.

Clinical management

Investigation

- Dementia blood screen – FBC, U&Es, LFTs, calcium, glucose, folate, B_{12} and TFTs.
- Urinalysis – to rule out UTI.
- MRI brain (or alternatively CT).

Explanation to patient

- Alzheimer's disease is the commonest type of dementia.
- It is caused by shrinkage of the brain, resulting in a reduction in the number of nerve fibres.
- The levels of some brain chemicals called neurotransmitters are also reduced, in particular acetylcholine, although the reason for this leading to memory problems is not clearly understood.
- Tiny deposits or plaques also form within the brain which can damage surrounding nerve cells. They can spread to the hippocampus part of the brain which is essential in forming memories.

Management

- Refer to memory clinic.
- Support and care from community teams, for example, district nurses, psychiatric teams, occupational therapy and social services.
- Physical activity and cognitive stimulation.
- Treat any risk factors for dementia, for example, smoking, excessive alcohol use, obesity, hypertension and high cholesterol.
- Medication – acetylcholinesterase inhibitors (e.g. donepezil, galantamine) in moderate Alzheimer's disease (MMSE score 10–20).
- Inform DVLA if still driving.
- Consider whether the patient has capacity to make decisions about their care. If the person lacks capacity, the provisions of the Mental Capacity Act 2005 must be followed (*NICE*, 2006, *CG42: Dementia*).
- Also consider the carer's needs.
- Safety net – if problems worsen to return to GP and also consider a regular review.

Role play

Information for doctor	Additional information for role player
Patient: Mrs WW *Age*: 83 years *SH*: Lives with husband. *PMH*: MI 1996, hypercholesterolaemia *DH*: Aspirin, simvastatin *Information*: You are a GP partner. Mr W has booked an appointment to chat about his wife.	*PC*: "*I am worried about my wife as she seems to be getting increasingly confused*" *HPC*: Was found wandering the streets last week. **Gets confused with where she is, and days of the week.** Still has good long-term memory. Last week she left her gas hob on. *ICE*: **Worried she may be developing Alzheimer's.** *O/E*: Neurological examination – NAD. MMSE – 14/30.

Falls

- Common presentation in the elderly, often with multi-factorial aetiology.
- Risk factors include visual impairment, cognitive impairment, muscle weakness, hypotension and poly-pharmacy.
- Management depends on the cause, although the NICE guidelines (2004, *CG21: Falls*) advise multi-factorial interventions.

Data gathering

Open question
- *"Can you tell me more about the falls you've been having?"*

Focused/closed questions

HPC: *"Do you know what is causing the falls?"*
"Have you ever lost consciousness?"
"Do you get any associated dizziness beforehand?"
Any triggers for the falls?
Were there any witnesses?
"Have you ever experienced the sensation of your heart pounding?"
"Have you ever lost control of your bladder?"

PMH: Any medical conditions?

FH: Any FH of osteoporosis or falls?

SH: *"Who lives with you at home?"* *"Do you have stairs at home?"* Support? Coping? Alcohol history?

DH: *"Are you on any regular medications?"* *"Do you take any blood pressure medications/sedatives?"*

Examination: (includes multifactorial falls risk assessment – *NICE*, 2004, *CG21: Falls*):
- BP, pulse.
- BMI.
- Cardiovascular system.
- Neurological examination including visual acuity, gait, mobility and balance.
- Mini mental state examination.

Clinical management

Investigations
- Blood test – FBC, U&Es, LFTs, TFTs, B_{12}, glucose.
- Urinalysis – check for leucocytes and nitrites.
- ECG.

Explanation to patient

- There are lots of different risk factors for falls. These include low body weight, being on medications such as beta-blockers and insulin, alcohol abuse, diabetes mellitus, confusion, and problems with vision or balance.
- There are various different measures which can be taken to help prevent falls.

Management

- Falls clinic.
- Prevention – stop any causative medications, strength and balance training, home hazard assessment and intervention, management of any visual problems, assess osteoporosis risk.
- Provide information leaflet about falls prevention.
- Safety net – arrange follow-up to assess progress.

Role play

Information for doctor	Additional information for role player
Patient: Mrs VH *Age*: 84 years *SH*: Lives in warden-controlled flat. *PMH*: Previous mitral valve repair 2006, hypertension, hypothyroidism. *DH*: Coracten, levothyroxine, aspirin *Information*: Was seen by the practice nurse for BP check last week (100/60 mmHg). Mentioned to nurse about recent history of falls. You are a salaried GP.	*PC*: Falls *HPC*: Has had several falls in recent weeks and the warden is quite concerned. Episodes of dizziness. **No syncope. No palpitations or SOB. No loss of consciousness. Warden witnessed one fall. Seemed to lose balance.** No known triggers. *ICE*: Warden concerned about the falls. *O/E*: Sitting BP 120/80 mmHg, standing BP 80/50 mmHg

Women's health

Menorrhagia

- Heavy periods, often defined as blood loss >80 mls.
- Cause is often not known, and this is referred to as 'dysfunctional uterine bleeding'.
- Other causes include fibroids, endometriosis, IUD *in situ* or hypothyroidism.
- Management includes LNG-IUS, tranexamic acid, COCP or surgical options.

Data gathering

Open question
- *"Can you tell me more about the heavy periods that you've been experiencing?"*

Focused/closed questions

HPC: *"When did the heavy periods first start?"*
"How many times do you change pads/tampons in a typical day?"
"Do you get any clots in the blood or any flooding?"
"Are your periods more painful than usual?"
"Do you get any abdominal pain or abdominal bloating?"
"Are your periods regular? When was your last menstrual period?"
"Do you get any bleeding in between your periods or after sex?" (red flag)
"Have you had a contraceptive coil fitted?"

PMH: Any other medical conditions? Any previous gynaecological surgery?

DH: *"Are you on any regular medications?"*

FH: Any conditions that run in the family?

ICE: *"Do you have any thoughts as to what might be causing the heavy bleeding?"*
"How is this problem affecting your day to day life?"

Examination:
- Abdominal/pelvic examination.
- Speculum examination.

Clinical management

Investigations
- Blood tests – FBC, ferritin, TFTs.

- Ultrasound scan of pelvis.
- Endometrial sampling.
- Hysteroscopy.

Explanation to patient

- Heavy periods often occur because the amount of a chemical called prostaglandin is increased in the lining of the womb.
- It can also be caused by fibroids (benign growths in the womb), endometriosis (endometrial tissue grows outside the womb) or a hormonal problem.

Management

- Menstrual diary.
- LNG-IUS – reduces heavy menstrual bleeding.
- Medications – tranexamic acid, COCP, norethisterone.
- Safety net – to see GP if problem not improving.
- Surgery – endometrial ablation, hysterectomy.

Role play

Information for doctor	Additional information for role player
Patient: Ms JE *Age:* 26 years *SH:* PhD student, lives with partner *PMH:* migraine *DH:* Nil *Information:* You are a GP Registrar.	*PC:* "I have been getting very heavy periods for the past 6 months" *HPC:* Changing tampons approx every 3 hours. **Has clots. No flooding.** Regular periods (LMP 2 weeks ago). Also gets quite severe abdominal pain during periods. **No discharge.** No other associated symptoms. **Has IUD *in situ*** (fitted 8 months ago) *ICE:* Would like some medication to help reduce the heavy bleeding. Also keen to know what is causing it. *O/E:* Abdominal examination – lower abdominal tenderness. Slight tenderness on PV examination.

Amenorrhoea

- Absence or cessation of menses, either classified as primary amenorrhoea (menses not occurring by the time of expected menarche) or secondary amenorrhoea (absence of menstruation for at least 6 consecutive months in women with previously normal and regular menses).
- Causes of primary amenorrhoea include constitutional delay, genito-urinary malformation, Turner syndrome and testicular feminisation.

- Causes of secondary amenorrhoea include hypothalamic failure, pregnancy and lactation, premature ovarian failure, weight loss, polycystic ovarian syndrome and depot or implant contraception.

Data gathering

Open question
- *"Can you tell me more about the problem with your periods?"*

Focused/closed questions

HPC: *"Have you ever had periods? If so, when was your last menstrual period?"*
"At what age did you start having periods (if secondary amenorrhoea)?"
"Is there any chance you could be pregnant?"
"Have there been any recent change in your weight or any increase in exercise?"
"Have you noticed any changes to your skin or hair?"
"Any lower abdominal pain?" (haematocolpos)
"Any hot flushes or vaginal dryness?" (menopause/premature ovarian failure)
"Have you ever had problems trying to get pregnant?"
"Any headache, problems with your vision or leakage of milk from your breasts?" (red flags)

PMH: Any medical conditions? PCOS? Thyroid problems? Depression? Previous surgery?

DH: *"Do you take any regular medications?"* Any hormonal contraceptives? Antipsychotics? Previous radiotherapy or chemotherapy?

FH: Any family history of menstrual problems? *"When did your mother and sister(s) start their periods?"*
Any family history of stopping periods before 40 years of age?

SH: Occupation/Studying? Stress? Who lives with you at home? Any problems? Illicit drug use, e.g. cocaine or opiates?

ICE: *"Do you have any thoughts as to why your periods might have stopped?"*

Examination (based on *NHS CKS*, 2009, *Amenorrhoea – management*):
- BMI.
- Examine for secondary sexual characteristics, e.g. Tanner Stages (N.B. no intimate examinations in the CSA).
- Examine for hirsutism, clitoromegaly, galactorrhoea and haematocolpos (if appropriate from history).
- Thyroid examination (if appropriate from history).
- Visual fields/fundoscopy (if pituitary tumour suspected).

Clinical management

Investigations
- Pregnancy test.
- Blood tests – serum LH, FSH, prolactin, TSH, testosterone, SHBG.
- Pelvic ultrasound scan.

Explanation to patient
- Amenorrhoea is the absence of menstrual periods in a woman of reproductive age.
- There may be a normal physiological explanation, for example, before puberty or due to pregnancy, breast-feeding or menopause, or it may be due to contraception, surgery or due to a medical condition.

Management (based on *NHS CKS*, 2009, *Amenorrhoea – management*)

Primary amenorrhoea
- Refer to a specialist any female who has not started menstruating by 14 years of age and has no secondary sexual characteristics, or females with normal secondary sexual characteristics who have not started menstruating by 16 years of age.

Secondary amenorrhoea
- Treat the underlying cause once the diagnosis is confirmed, e.g. counselling if stress induced or stopping any causative drugs.
- Refer to a specialist if the cause cannot be established or if treatment in secondary care is required.
- The following conditions can usually be managed in primary care – PCOS, menopause and amenorrhoea due to weight loss, stress or exercise.
- Manage the risk of osteoporosis.
- Safety net – if not resolving to return to GP.

Role play

Information for doctor	Additional information for role player
Patient: Ms SL *Age*: 17 years *SH*: College student, lives with parents *PMH*: Acne *DH*: Nil *Information*: consultation with locum GP 2 weeks ago – tiredness, weight gain. TFTs checked and normal. BMI 34. You are a GP partner.	*PC*: "*I have not had a period for the past 8 months*". *HPC*: Previously had periods. Started menstruating aged 12 years. Also increased facial hair. No skin changes. No headache or visual problems. *ICE*: **Worried about being pregnant. Hoping for a pregnancy test.** Pregnancy test – negative. Evidence of hirsutism.

Premenstrual syndrome

- Condition in which women experience certain symptoms each month before their menstrual period.
- Most commonly affects women aged between 30 and 40 years.
- Symptoms may be physical (e.g. breast tenderness, bloating, headaches) and/or psychological (e.g. tension, irritability, low mood, loss of libido).
- Treatments include SSRIs, COCP or CBT.

Data gathering

Open question
- *"Can you describe the symptoms you experience prior to your period?"*

Focused/closed questions

HPC: *"Do you suffer with any breast tenderness, bloating or headaches prior to your period?"*
"Do you experience any mood changes prior to your period?"
"Have you noticed any changes to your sex drive?"
"How long have you been experiencing these symptoms?"
"How long do they last for each time?"
"Have you tried anything so far to relieve the symptoms?"

PMH: Any history of depression or any other medical conditions?

DH: *"Do you take any regular medications?"*

FH: Any family history of PMS?

SH: Occupation? Who lives with you at home? Smoking/alcohol/illicit drug history?

ICE: *"How have the symptoms been affecting your day to day life?"*

Examination: • Nothing specific.

Clinical management

Investigations
- Symptom diary.

Explanation to patient
- PMS is quite a common problem, although it is only bad enough to affect daily life in about 1 in 20 women.
- There is no test for PMS and it is diagnosed purely on the symptoms described.
- The cause is not known, although ovulation with the release of an egg appears to trigger symptoms.

Management (based on *RCOG, 2007, Green-top guideline 48: Management of premenstrual syndrome*)

- General advice about exercise, diet and stress reduction.
- Medications, e.g. SSRI or COCP.
- CBT.
- Information leaflet.
- Safety net – refer to gynaecologist when simple measures have been explored but have failed.

Role play

Information for doctor	Additional information for role player
Patient: Ms TB *Age*: 21 years *SH*: University student. *FH*: Nil *PMH*: Nil *DH*: Nil *Information*: You are a GP partner. Temporary patient.	*PC*: *"I have terrible mood swings around the time of my period".* *HPC*: *"Something needs to be done because I got into trouble in a night club as I got aggressive towards someone".* Also broke up with boyfriend because of aggression/mood. Gets occasional breast tenderness and bloating. No headaches. *ICE*: **Needs some medication to take around her periods to help with mood.**

Polycystic ovary syndrome

- Condition resulting in tiny cysts forming on the ovaries (at least 12 cysts).
- Can result in abnormal periods, reduced fertility, excessive hair growth and acne.
- Exact cause is unclear, but could be hereditary or linked to insulin resistance and/or obesity.
- Treatment depends on the symptoms, but includes weight loss, metformin and/or hormonal contraception to regulate periods.
- The figure opposite shows how you could illustrate polycystic ovaries to your patient.

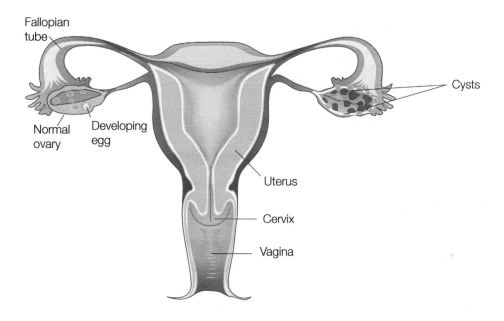

Data gathering

Open questions
- *"What do you know about polycystic ovary syndrome?"*
- *"Can you tell me more about your symptoms?"*

Focused/closed questions

HPC: *"When was your last menstrual period?"*
"Are your periods regular? Have there been any changes in your periods recently?"
"Do you get any abdominal pain?"
"Have you noticed any skin changes or excessive hair growth?"
"Have there been any changes in your mood?"
"Have there been any changes in your weight?"
"Any problems trying to get pregnant?"

FH: Any family history of PCOS?

SH Smoking/alcohol/illicit drug history? Occupation? Stress?

ICE: *"Was there anything in particular you were concerned about with these symptoms?"*

Examination:
- BMI.
- BP.
- Pelvic examination.

Clinical management

Investigations

- Blood test – total and free testosterone, SHBG, free androgen index, prolactin, TSH*.
- Pregnancy test (if appropriate).
- Pelvic ultrasound scan.

*LH and FSH are not routinely recommended for diagnosis of PCOS, but may help to rule out other causes (*RCOG*, 2007, *Green-top guideline 33: Long term consequences of polycystic ovary syndrome*) .

Explanation to patient

- PCOS is a condition which can affect a woman's menstrual cycle, fertility, hormones and aspects of her appearance. It can also affect long-term health.
- Cysts develop on the ovaries which results in an imbalance of the hormones produced by the ovaries.
- The ovaries produce more testosterone which can result in excessive hair growth and acne. The hormones released by the ovary are responsible for controlling the menstrual cycle and so this can also be affected.
- Some patients may no longer ovulate which will result in fertility problems.

Management

- Lifestyle changes – weight loss and healthy balanced diet.
- Metformin.
- Dianette.
- Other hormonal contraceptives to regulate periods.
- Eflornithine – for hirsutism.
- Clomifene – if fertility problems.
- Safety net – refer to a specialist if the above measures are not improving symptoms.

Role play

Information for doctor	Additional information for role player
Patient: Ms SS *Age*: 23 years *PMH*: Nil *DH*: Nil *Information*: Saw locum GP 1 month ago due to secondary amenorrhoea and hirsutism. USS of pelvis confirms polycystic ovaries. You are a GP Registrar.	*PC*: "*I have come today to get the results of my ultrasound scan*." *HPC*: LMP 8 months ago. Has noticed increased facial hair. **No skin changes. No other gynaecological symptoms. Never tried to conceive.** *FH*: **Sister has PCOS.** *ICE*: Thinks that she might also have PCOS. Would like medication to get rid of the increased facial hair. *O/E*: BMI – 34.

Fibroids

- Benign growths in the uterus.
- Very common, affecting at least 1 in 4 women in their lifetime.
- Commonest in the 30–50 year age group and in Afro–Caribbean women.
- Can be treated with medication, LNG-IUS or with surgery.
- The figure below shows how you could illustrate fibroids to your patient.

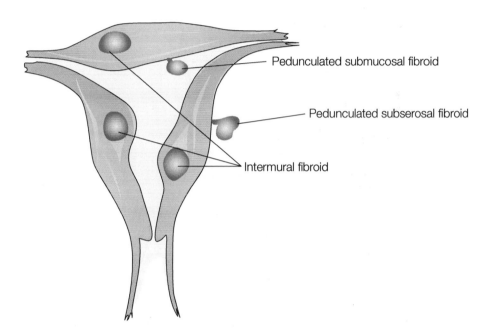

Pedunculated submucosal fibroid

Pedunculated subserosal fibroid

Intermural fibroid

Data gathering

Open questions
- *"Can you tell me more about your symptoms?"*
- *"The recent ultrasound scan you had has confirmed fibroids: what do you know about fibroids?"*

Closed/focused questions
HPC: *"Are your periods regular?"*
  "Are your periods heavier than usual?"
  "Any bleeding in between your periods or after sex?" (red flags)
  "Have you noticed any abdominal pain or swelling?"

"*Do you have any urinary symptoms?*"

"*Has there been any weight loss?*" (red flag)

FH: Any family history of fibroids?

SH: Smoking/alcohol/illicit drug history? Occupation?

ICE: "*What were you hoping we could do to help with your symptoms?*"

Examination:
- Abdominal examination.
- Vaginal examination.
- Speculum examination.

Clinical management

Investigations
- Pelvic ultrasound scan.
- FBC – if concerned about anaemia.
- Hysteroscopy or laparoscopy – in secondary care.

Explanation to patient
- Fibroids are non-cancerous growths which form in the womb, usually as a result of an overgrowth of smooth muscle cells.
- They can cause symptoms such as heavy bleeding, abdominal swelling and urinary problems.
- They can increase or decrease in size with time. During pregnancy they often increase in size due to the increased level of a hormone called oestrogen.

Management
- Observation and safety net – if symptoms not improving return to GP.
- Medication – tranexamic acid, NSAIDs, COCP, GnRH analogue to shrink the fibroids.
- LNG-IUS.
- Non-surgical treatments – endometrial ablation, uterine artery embolisation.
- Surgery – hysterectomy, myomectomy.

Role play

Information for doctor	Additional information for role player
Patient: Mrs JS Age: 34 years PMH: Nil DH: Ibuprofen Information: Recently seen by locum GP due to abdominal pain and menorrhagia. Results of pelvic USS – numerous fibroids visible in endometrium. Largest 5 cm x 4 cm diameter. You are a GP partner.	PC: "*I was asked to come in to discuss the results of my pelvic ultrasound scan*". HPC: Lower abdominal pain for the past couple of months. Also heavy periods. LMP 2 weeks ago. Regular periods. No urinary symptoms. ICE: **Worried she might have cancer.** O/E: Lower abdominal tenderness. Abdomen soft. PV exam – NAD.

Antenatal check

- All pregnant women in the UK are offered a series of antenatal appointments during their pregnancy.
- In the case of an uncomplicated pregnancy, this care should be provided by midwives and GPs (*NICE*, 2008, *CG62: Antenatal care*).
- In an uncomplicated pregnancy, nulliparous women are offered 10 antenatal appointments, and parous women are offered 7 appointments.
- The first booking appointment is around 10–12 weeks.
- The antenatal checks include weight, blood pressure, urine dipstick for protein, glucose and leucocytes, and blood tests for blood group, rhesus group and infections.
- The growth of the baby is checked using symphysis–fundal height (SFH), and the position of the baby is also checked in the later stages of pregnancy.
- Ultrasound scans are carried out at 12 and 20 weeks gestation, and Down syndrome screening is also offered.

Data gathering

Open question
- *"How is the pregnancy going so far?"*

Focused/closed questions

HPC: *"When was your last menstrual period?"*
"When is your expected date of delivery?"
"Have you felt any kicks or the baby moving?"
"Do you have any ankle swelling?"
"Are you getting any abdominal pains?"
"Have you noticed any vaginal bleeding?"

PMH: *"Do you suffer from any medical conditions?"*

DH: Do you take any regular medications?
"Have you been taking folic acid?"

SH: Who lives with you at home? Support? Occupation? Smoking/alcohol/illicit drug history?

ICE: *"Do you have any concerns about the pregnancy?"*

Examination: • See clinical management.

Clinical management (based on *NICE*, 2008, *CG62: Antenatal care*)

First contact with a healthcare professional
- Provide information on folic acid supplements, lifestyle advice and antenatal screening.

Lifestyle advice

- Smoking cessation – nicotine replacement therapy can be used in pregnancy.
- Alcohol consumption – avoid alcohol in the first 3 months if at all possible. If women choose to drink alcohol, drink no more than 1–2 units of alcohol once or twice a week.
- Folic acid supplement prior to conception until 12 weeks gestation – 400 mcg daily (or 5 mg daily if your risk of having a child with a neural tube defect is increased).
- Vitamin D supplements during pregnancy and breast-feeding if inadequate stores – 10 mcg daily.
- Give dietary advice to reduce risk of listeriosis, salmonella and toxoplasmosis.
- Advise on which drugs to avoid, e.g. NSAIDs.

Booking appointment

- Identify women who may need additional care.
- Calculate BMI.
- Measure BP and check urine for proteinuria and bacteriuria.
- Offer blood test for blood group, rhesus D status, FBC, haemoglobinopathies, Hep B, HIV, rubella immunity and syphilis.
- Offer screening for Down syndrome.
- Offer ultrasound scans for gestational age assessment at 12 weeks and to check for any fetal anomalies at 20 weeks.
- Inform women under 25 years about the national chlamydia screening programme.
- Determine if any risk factors for gestational diabetes or pre-eclampsia.
- Inform women about maternity benefits available.

25 weeks (nulliparous women)

- Measure BP and check urine for proteinuria.
- Measure symphysis–fundal height.

28–34 weeks

- Check SFH.
- Offer further screening for anaemia.
- Offer anti-D prophylaxis for those women who are rhesus D negative.
- Discuss a birth plan.

36–38 weeks

- Check position of baby, and refer for external cephalic version if breech.
- Discuss breast-feeding and postnatal care.

41 weeks

- If not yet given birth, refer for membrane sweep and induction of labour.

Role play

Information for doctor	Additional information for role player
Patient: Mrs SC *Age*: 32 years *PMH*: Nil *DH*: Nil *Information*: Has appointment today for routine 30 week antenatal check. You are a GP Registrar.	*HPC*: Currently 30 weeks pregnant. Hasn't felt baby moving for the past 2 days. No vaginal bleeding or abdominal pain. First pregnancy. *ICE*: **No real concerns although a bit worried that she hasn't felt fetal movements.** *O/E*: SFH 26 cm, no fetal heart sounds heard.

Urinary incontinence

- Involuntary leakage of urine, estimated to affect about 3 million people in the UK.
- Different types include stress, urge, mixed and overflow incontinence.
- Management includes lifestyle changes, pelvic floor exercises, bladder training or medication.

Data gathering

Open question
- "Can you tell me more about the problems with your bladder?"

Closed/focused questions

HPC: *"How often do you lose control of your bladder?" "Is it only when coughing or sneezing, or does it occur at any time?"*
"Have you tried any treatments so far?"
"Do you suffer with frequent urine infections?"
"Do you have any burning pain when you pass urine?"
"Have you noticed any blood in the urine or vaginal bleeding?" (red flag)
"Have you noticed a lump coming down from your vagina?"
"Do you have any problems with your bowels?"
"Have you noticed any weight loss?" (red flag)

DH: Do you take any regular medications? Diuretics?

FH: Any family history of bladder problems?

SH: Smoking/alcohol/illicit drug history? Occupation?

PMH: Any previous operations?

ICE: *"How is this problem impacting on your daily life?"*

Examination:
- Abdominal examination.
- Digital rectal examination.
- Sims speculum examination to check for prolapse.

Clinical management

Investigations

- Urinalysis – blood, glucose, protein, leucocytes, nitrites.
- Urodynamics (only after conservative management).

Explanation to patient

- There are different types of urinary incontinence:
  - Stress incontinence occurs when the pressure in the bladder becomes too great and urine leaks from the bladder outlet. This is often due to the pelvic floor muscles being weak.
  - Urge incontinence is when you get an urgent desire to pass urine and are unable to get to the toilet in time. It's often due to a problem with the bladder muscles sending wrong messages to the brain.
  - Mixed incontinence is a combination of stress and urge incontinence.
  - Overflow incontinence is due to an obstruction of the outflow of urine.

Management (*NICE*, 2006, *CG40: Urinary incontinence*)

- Lifestyle modifications – weight loss, modify fluid intake and decrease caffeine and alcohol intake.
- Bladder diary for minimum of 3 days.
- Pelvic floor muscle training for minimum of 3 months – first line treatment for stress or mixed incontinence.
- Bladder training for minimum of 6 weeks – first line treatment for urge or mixed incontinence.
- Medications – oxybutynin first line for overactive bladder or mixed incontinence (alternative is solifenacin).
- Refer to secondary care for surgical management if conservative management hasn't helped or if there is a symptomatic prolapse visible at or below the vaginal introitus.
- Urgently refer if microscopic haematuria and aged 50 years or over, visible haematuria, suspected pelvic mass arising from the urinary tract or recurrent or persistent UTI associated with haematuria in those aged 40 years or older.

Role play

Information for doctor	Additional information for role player
Patient: Mrs JW *Age*: 47 years *SH*: Married, has 3 children. *PMH*: Nil *DH*: Nil *Information*: No recent consultations. You are a GP partner.	*PC*: Urinary incontinence *HPC*: Has urinary incontinence intermittently but it is becoming more frequent. **Occurs mainly after coughing, sneezing or exercise. No blood in the urine. No abdominal pain. No prolapse. No pain when passing urine. Not tried any treatments so far. Two urine infections in the past year.** *ICE*: Has heard about surgery to help this problem and is keen to find out more. *O/E*: Abdominal examination – NAD.

Cervical screening

- Offered to all women aged between 25 and 65 in England and Northern Ireland (20–65 years in Scotland and Wales).
- The aim is to detect any pre-cancerous cells.
- The screening is carried out 3-yearly from 20 or 25 years to 50 years and then 5-yearly until aged 65.

Data gathering

Open question
- *"What do you understand about an abnormal cervical smear result?"*

Focused/closed questions

HPC: *"Have you had any irregular menstrual bleeding?"*
"Have you had any bleeding in between your periods or after sex?" (red flags)
"Have you noticed any abnormal discharge?"
"Do you have any abdominal pain?"
"Have you recently noticed any weight loss?" (red flag)

FH: Any family history of cervical cancer?

SH: *"Do you smoke?"* Who lives with you at home? Occupation?

ICE: *"Did you have any specific concerns about your smear test result?"*

Examination: • Liquid cervical smear test via speculum examination.

Clinical management

Investigations
- Refer for colposcopy if moderate or severe dyskaryosis or two consecutive results showing mild dyskaryosis.

Explanation to patient
- Cells are gently scraped from the neck of the womb using a plastic brush.
- These cells are then sent to the lab to be examined under a microscope.
- If there are any abnormal cells seen, you may be referred for a colposcopy.
- A colposcopy is a detailed examination of the cervix using an instrument called a colposcope. It allows a more detailed view of any abnormal cells in the cervix, and a further sample of tissue can be taken if necessary.
- If the colposcopy reveals an abnormal result, you may need further treatment to remove or destroy the abnormal cells in your cervix. This can be done using laser treatment or by cutting out the affected area. If there are only mild changes in the cervix, the abnormal cells may return to normal on their own.

Management

- Smoking cessation.
- Treatment for abnormal cells include cryotherapy, loop diathermy, laser treatment or cold coagulation (organised by gynaecologist).
- Safety net – review if symptoms worsen and arrange follow-up smear tests.
- Information – www.cancerscreening.nhs.uk/cervical.

Role play

Information for doctor	Additional information for role player
Patient: Ms TS *Age*: 27 years *SH*: Single, lives alone, smoker, 15 units alcohol/wk *FH*: Mum has breast cancer. *Information*: Had smear test done 4 weeks ago. Results – moderate dyskaryosis. You are a GP Partner.	*PC*: "I was asked to come in to discuss my cervical smear results" *HPC*: Has had intermenstrual and some post-coital bleeding for past few months. **No abdo pain. No weight loss. LMP 1 week ago. No previous abnormal smear tests. Last smear test 3 years ago.** *ICE*: **Worried about why she was called to come in.** Worried that she might have cervical cancer because of the symptoms.

Infertility

- Failure to conceive after regular unprotected intercourse for 2 years in the absence of known reproductive pathology (*NICE*, 2004, *CG11: Fertility*).
- Approximately 1 in 7 couples have difficulty conceiving.

Data gathering

Open question

- "Can you tell me more about your problems trying to get pregnant?"

Focused/closed questions

HPC: "When was your last menstrual period?" "Are your periods regular?"
"Have you noticed any bleeding in between your periods or after intercourse?" (red flag)
"Do you have any abdominal pain?"
"How often are you having intercourse?"
"When did you stop using any contraception?"
"Have you ever been pregnant before?"
"Has your partner had any children before?"
Take a full sexual history – see *Appendix 2*.

PMH: Any medical conditions? Any history of pelvic inflammatory disease, endometriosis or ectopic pregnancy? Any previous gynaecological surgery? Any history of depression?

SH: Who lives with you at home? Occupation? Stress? Alcohol/smoking/illicit drug history?

FH: Any family history of fertility problems?

DH: Do you take any regular medications? Any over the counter medications?

ICE: *"Do you have any thoughts as to why you are having difficulties conceiving?"*

Examination: • BMI.
• Vaginal and speculum examination.
• Abdominal examination.

Clinical management

Investigations

- Blood tests – day 21 progesterone, serum LH and FSH (if irregular menstrual cycle).
- Semen analysis ($\male$).
- Screen for chlamydia before undergoing any uterine instrumentation.
- Rubella screening.
- Pelvic ultrasound scan if indicated from history.

Explanation to patient

- It is important to be reassured that 84% of all couples will conceive within 1 year if they do not use contraception and have regular intercourse.
- There are various different reasons for fertility problems, some of which are related to the man and some to the woman. Further tests can help to establish the cause.
- There are options to help which include advice about lifestyle changes, medications and referral to a fertility specialist.

Management (*NICE, 2004, CG11: Fertility*)

- Lifestyle advice – smoking cessation, reduce alcohol intake, healthy diet, weight loss, exercise.
- Sexual intercourse every 2–3 days optimises the chance of pregnancy.
- Folic acid supplements.
- Fertility support group.
- Counselling.
- Refer to fertility clinic for further investigations/management if not pregnant after 1 year despite above measures.
  - Women with ovulation disorders such as PCOS should be offered clomifene citrate as first line to induce ovulation.

○ Couples in which the woman is aged between 23 and 39 years at the time of treatment, and who have an identifiable cause for their fertility problems, or who have had infertility for at least 3 years duration should be offered up to three stimulated cycles of *in vitro* fertilisation. Unfortunately, due to financial pressures, one in five PCTs have reduced the number of treatment cycles that they are able to offer.

Role play

Information for doctor	Additional information for role player
Patient: Mrs KS *Age*: 32 years *PMH*: Nil *DH*: Nil *Information*: No previous consultations. You are a GP Registrar.	*PC*: "*I've been trying to get pregnant for the past 14 months and it hasn't worked*" *HPC*: **Never been pregnant before.** Partner has never had children. Having unprotected sex 4x weekly. LMP 3 weeks ago. Regular periods. No abdominal pain. *SH*: Married 3 years ago. Lives with husband and husband's sister. Accountant. Stressful job. Non-smoker, 5 units alcohol/week. *ICE*: **Worried about why she can't conceive and wants referral to fertility specialist.** *O/E*: BMI – 23. Abdominal and vaginal exam – NAD.

Menopause

- Permanent cessation of ovarian function, typically occurring around the age of 50 years.
- A woman has reached menopause when she has not had a period for one year.
- If menopause occurs under the age of 45 years it is known as premature menopause.

Data gathering

Open question
- "Can you tell me more about the menopausal symptoms you have been experiencing?"

Focused/closed questions
HPC: "*When was your last menstrual period?*"
"*Have you noticed any changes to your periods?*"
"*Have you experienced any hot flushes, night sweats or headaches?*"
"*Have you noticed any mood changes, loss of sex drive or difficulty sleeping?*"
"*Have you noticed any vaginal dryness?*"

"Any abdominal pain or swelling of the abdomen?" (red flag)
"Any bleeding at least 1 year after your periods had stopped?" (red flags)

SH: Smoking/alcohol/illicit drug history? Who lives with you at home? Occupation?

ICE: *"Are these symptoms affecting your day to day life?"*

Examination: • BP.

Clinical management

Investigations
- Blood test – LH, FSH, oestrogen.

Explanation to patient
- The menopause naturally occurs when the ovaries stop producing eggs and this results in lower levels of the female hormone oestrogen.
- Various symptoms can occur including mood changes, hot flushes and changes to the vagina and genital skin. For some people these symptoms can be quite debilitating, and treatment is required to help alleviate these symptoms.

Management (based on *NHS CKS*, 2008, *Menopause – evidence*)
- Lifestyle changes – healthy diet, exercise.
- HRT
  - Usually oestrogen/progesterone combined, or oestrogen only if previous hysterectomy
  - Preparations include tablets, patches and gels
  - Different types include cyclical combined and continuous combined:
    - cyclical combined is suitable for those still experiencing erratic menstrual bleeding. Oestrogen is taken daily, and progesterone is added for the last 12–14 days of the cycle. You will continue to get monthly periods.
    - continuous combined preparations are used once a woman has not had a natural period for at least a year. It involves a daily dose of oestrogen and progesterone and you will not get monthly bleeds.
  - Benefits include reducing symptoms of hot flushes and may protect against osteoporosis
  - Disadvantages include small increased risk of breast cancer, DVT and endometrial cancer.
- Tibolone – synthetic steroid hormone which helps with hot flushes, sweats and vaginal dryness.
- Clonidine – relieves hot flushes.
- Vaginal lubricants
- SSRIs – effective for hot flushes (not licensed).
- Safety net – if no improvement in symptoms return to GP. Patients on HRT should be followed up 3 months after starting treatment, and yearly thereafter.

Role play

Information for doctor	Additional information for role player
Patient: Ms PO *Age*: 54 years *SH*: Lives alone, school teacher. Non-smoker. *PMH*: Breast cancer *DH*: Tamoxifen *Information*: Last saw GP 1 month ago for medication review. You are a locum GP.	*PC*: Menopausal symptoms *HPC*: Experiencing bad hot flushes and some mood swings and vaginal dryness. LMP 8 months ago. **Also has problems sleeping.** *FH*: **Breast cancer (sister).** *ICE*: Would like to know what she could take to help with her menopausal symptoms.

Men's health

Benign prostatic hypertrophy

- Benign prostatic hypertrophy (BPH) refers to prostate gland enlargement, which can often cause problems with passing urine.
- Common in older men.
- The figure below shows how you could illustrate the prostate to your patient.

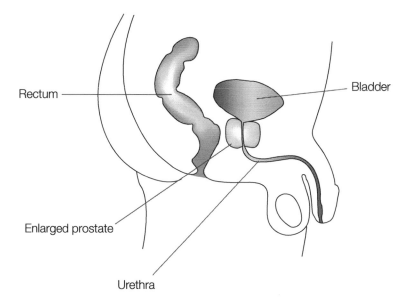

Data gathering

Open question
- *"Do you mind telling me more about your urinary symptoms?"*

Focused/closed questions
HPC: *"Have you been passing urine more frequently than normal? Have you had to rush to get to the toilet to pass urine? Have you had any hesitancy when trying to pass urine, or has the stream of urine been poor?"*

"Do you have any dribbling at the end of the stream of urine? Have you ever been unable to pass urine?"

"Do you wake up at night to pass urine?" " If so, how many times?"

"Have you noticed any weight loss, bone pains or blood in the urine?" (red flags)

PMH: Do you suffer with any other medical conditions?

DH: Do you take any regular medications? Diuretics?

SH: Smoking/alcohol/illicit drug history? Occupation?

FH: Any family history of bladder problems?

ICE: *"Do you have any particular worries/concerns about your bladder symptoms?".*

Examination:
- Prostate examination (offer chaperone).
- Abdominal examination – check bladder and kidneys.

Clinical management

Investigations
- Urine dipstick – check for haematuria.
- Blood test – PSA and U&Es.
- Voiding diary.

Explanation to patient
- The prostate gland is found beneath the bladder and is approximately the size of a chestnut. It is only found in men.
- The prostate gland produces fluid which protects and enriches sperm.
- A tube-like structure called the urethra carries urine from the bladder and this runs through the middle of the prostate. The urethra can be narrowed if the prostate enlarges and this is what causes the urinary symptoms.

Management (NICE, 2010, CG97: Lower urinary tract infections)
- Conservative management – watch and wait.
- Double voiding.
- Reduce intake of caffeine and alcohol.
- Bladder training.
- Stop smoking.
- Drug treatment:
  - Alpha-blockers, e.g. tamsulosin (relaxes smooth muscle of the prostate).
  - 5-alpha reductase inhibitors, e.g. finasteride (blocks the conversion of an enzyme in the prostate that is responsible for prostatic enlargement.
- Surgery – TURP (transurethral resection of the prostate) or prostatectomy.
- Safety net – if symptoms not improving return to GP.

Role play

Information for doctor	Additional information for role player
Patient: Mr SJ *Age*: 70 years *SH*: Retired, lives alone. Widowed *PMH*: Hypertension *FH*: Nil *DH*: Ramipril *Information*: You are a locum GP in the practice.	*PC*: Urinary problems for the past 4 months. *HPC*: Some terminal dribbling and incomplete emptying. No urgency. **No haematuria, weight loss or bone pains. Wakes up 3 x at night to pass urine.** *ICE*: Worried about prostate cancer as a close friend died from this. *O/E*: Smooth enlarged prostate gland

Prostate cancer

- Cancer which develops from cells in the prostate gland.
- Commonest cancer in men in the UK according to Cancer Research UK (2007, *Prostate cancer – UK incidence statistics*).
- Many cases are slow growing and may not affect life expectancy.

Data gathering

Open question

- *"Do you mind telling me more about the problems with your bladder symptoms?"*

Focused/closed questions

HPC: *"Have you been passing urine more frequently than usual? Have you had any difficulties passing urine?"*

"Do you ever have to rush to get to the toilet on time? Do you ever have any dribbling at the end of passing urine or a poor urine stream?"

"Do you wake up at night to pass urine?" "If so, how many times?"

"Have you passed any blood in the urine? Any pain when passing urine? Have you ever been unable to pass urine or not been able to empty your bladder fully?"

"Do you have any erectile problems?"

"Have you noticed any weight loss or bone pain?" (red flags)

PMH: Do you suffer with any other medical conditions?

DH: Do you take any regular medications?

SH: Smoking/alcohol/drug history? Occupation? Who lives with you at home?

FH: Any family history of prostate cancer or bladder problems?

ICE: *"What did you think might be causing your symptoms?"*

"Did you have any particular worries/concerns about your urinary symptoms?"

Examination: • Prostate examination.
• Abdominal examination – for palpation of enlarged bladder.

Clinical management

Investigations
- Urine dipstick (check for haematuria).
- PSA test (see www.nice.org.uk/nicemedia/live/11924/39524/39524.pdf).
- Biopsy of the prostate (done by urologist).

Explanation to patient
- Cells in the prostate (see also *Figure 4*) become abnormal and they multiply 'out of control'.
- Mostly occurs in men over the age of 65 years.
- Risk factors include ageing, family history, ethnicity (commoner in Afro–Caribbean men), diet, environmental factors.

Management
- Refer under 2 week wait cancer referral if suspected prostate cancer.
- Active surveillance and safety net.
- Surgery – radical prostatectomy.
- Radiotherapy or chemotherapy.
- Hormone treatment, e.g. goserelin.

N.B. Screening for prostate cancer is controversial (see *PSA testing* for further information).

Role play

Information for doctor	Additional information for role player
Patient: Mr JE *Age:* 65 years *SH:* Retired, lives with wife. Smokes 10 cigs/day *PMH:* Hypercholesterolaemia *DH:* Simvastatin 40 mg OD. *Information:* Saw a GP partner last week due to haematuria, urgency and frequency. Came today for PSA result which is 16 ng/ml. You are a salaried GP.	*PC:* Urinary symptoms. *HPC:* Haematuria, urgency and frequency for the past 6 months. 5 kg weight loss in past 4 months. **No incomplete emptying or terminal dribbling. No bone pain/dysuria/erectile problems.** *ICE:* **Thinks his symptoms are due to 'old age'. Not worried about cancer. Hoping for medication to alleviate his symptoms.**

PSA testing

Information for patients
- Blood test that measures the level of prostate specific antigen (PSA) in the blood.
- The PSA is produced by the prostate and is raised in certain conditions, for example: a raised PSA can be a sign of prostate cancer, or BPH, or urinary infection, or a response to a recent examination of the prostate, recent biopsy of the prostate, or the result of exercise.
- Two out of three people with a raised PSA will not have prostate cancer.
- If the PSA result is not raised, it is unlikely to be prostate cancer.
- If the PSA result is mildly elevated, the patient probably doesn't have cancer, but should be monitored.
- If the PSA is very elevated, the patient should be referred to urology following a prostate examination.
- Normal PSA values are generally considered to be <3 ng/ml in those under 60, <4 ng/ml in those aged 60–69 and <5 ng/ml in those over 70.
- Offer patients the following information sheet: www.cancerscreening.nhs.uk/prostate/prostate-patient-info-sheet.pdf

Testicular cancer

- Cancer of the testes accounts for just 1% of all male cancers.
- 50% of cases are under 35 years old.
- Risk factors include family history, undescended testes, mumps and possibly environmental factors.
- Curable in 95% of cases.

Data gathering

Open question
- "Can you tell me more about this testicular lump/swelling that you have noticed?"

Focused/closed questions
HPC: "When did you first notice the lump in your testicle?"
"Is it painful?"
"Has the lump increased in size recently?"
"Do you have any pain or discomfort in the groin?"
"Do you have any urinary symptoms?"
"Have you noticed any weight loss or bone pains?" (red flags)
"Do you have any shortness of breath or are you coughing up blood?" (red flags)

PMH: Any history of undescended testes? Any history of mumps?

FH: Any family history of testicular problems?

SH: Occupation? Smoking/alcohol history?

ICE: *"Was there anything in particular you were concerned about?"*
"How have these symptoms been affecting you?"

Examination: • Testicular examination (offer chaperone).
• Abdominal examination.
• Examine lymph nodes.

Clinical management

Investigations

- Scrotal ultrasound scan.
- Blood test for tumour markers (AFP, HCG, LDH).

Explanation to patient

- The testes are the two male sex organs that sit inside the scrotum.
- They produce sperm and the hormone testosterone which is important in male sexual development.
- The cells that become cancerous are those that are involved in making the sperm.

Management

- Refer to urologist under 2 week rule if suspected testicular cancer.
- Surgery and/or chemotherapy/radiotherapy if proven testicular cancer.
- Encourage health promotion – regular testicular examinations.
- Safety net – if symptoms worsen or are not improving return to GP.

Role play

Information for doctor	Additional information for role player
Patient: Mr IK *Age*: 24 years old *SH*: University student, single, lives with 2 friends. Non smoker, no alcohol. *PMH*: Undescended testes. *DH*: Nil *Information*: You are a salaried GP.	*PC*: Testicular swelling *HPC*: Noticed testicular swelling 4 weeks ago. Not worsened since then. Painless swelling. No groin discomfort/pain. **No haematuria. No urinary symptoms. No weight loss.** *FH*: Nil. *ICE*: Unsure what is causing his symptoms. *O/E*: Discrete firm testicular mass palpable in left testis.

Erectile dysfunction

- Impotence is the inability to get and/or maintain an erection.

Causes to consider

- Blood vessel narrowing secondary to hypertension, smoking, diabetes, or hypercholesterolaemia.
- Psychological causes, e.g. stress, anxiety, depression.
- Medication – e.g. beta-blockers, anti-depressants, cimetidine.
- Neurological causes, e.g. multiple sclerosis, stroke or spinal injury.
- Alcohol and drug abuse.
- Radiotherapy treatment to the pelvis.
- Hormonal causes.

Data gathering

Open question

- *"Can you tell me a bit more about the erectile problems you've been having?"*

Focused/closed questions

HPC: *"How long has the problem been going on for?" "Is it getting worse?" "Are you ever able to get an erection?" "Do you get early morning erections?"*
"Do you have any urinary problems?"
"Have you noticed any blood in your urine?" (red flag)

PMH: Any history of any medical conditions (e.g. prostate cancer, diabetes, hypertension, neurological problems or depression)?

DH: Any regular medications, e.g. beta-blockers?

SH: Smoking/alcohol/illicit drugs history? Are you in a stable relationship? Any problems with your relationship? Have you had any other sexual partners recently? If so, do you also have erectile problems with this partner? Occupation?

ICE: *"Do you have any idea what might be causing the erectile problems?"*
"How is this problem affecting you in terms of your relationship?"

Examination:
- BMI.
- Blood pressure.
- Prostate examination if relevant history.

Clinical management

Investigations

- Blood test – fasting glucose and cholesterol, U&Es, PSA.

Explanation to patient

- Erectile dysfunction is usually caused by poor blood flow to the penis.
- The commonest reason for this is narrowing of the blood vessels due to formation of fatty plaques called atheromas.
- Psychological reasons are other common causes of erectile dysfunction.
- Smoking and alcohol are common risk factors.
- Various different medical conditions and medications can also predispose to erectile problems, for example diabetes, high blood pressure, beta-blockers and anti-depressant medications.

Management

- Lifestyle advice (smoking cessation, healthy diet, exercise).
- If possible psychiatric cause, consider counselling, reducing stress levels and/or anti-depressants.
- If related to medication consider stopping the medication or changing to an alternative.
- Medication – sildenafil, tadalafil (work by increasing blood flow to the penis); these are only available on a private script unless the patient has a specific medical condition which qualifies for NHS prescription (see www.bnf.org).
- Injection therapy, vacuum devices, penile prosthesis.
- Patient information leaflet – www.patient.co.uk/health/Erectile-Dysfunction-(Impotence).htm.
- Safety net – if not improving after 4–6 weeks return to GP.

Role play

Information for doctor	Additional information for role player
Patient: Mr DG *Age*: 48 years old *SH*: Accountant, married with 2 children. *DH*: Nil *PMH*: Nil *FH*: Diabetes *Information*: You are a GP Registrar. This patient has never been seen in the surgery before.	*PC*: Erectile problems. *HPC*: Four month history of difficulty getting and maintaining erection. **Gets early morning erections. Marriage problems for past 6 months.** Feels low in mood. Poor sleep. Stress at work. *ICE*: **Very worried that these erectile problems are exacerbating the problems with his marriage.** Keen to have Viagra to improve things.

Testicular conditions

- Possible testicular conditions include hydrocoele, varicocoele and epididymo-orchitis.

Hydrocoele
- Collection of fluid in the scrotal sac around the testes.
- Usually unilateral but can be bilateral.
- Normally painless.
- Trans-illuminates on examination.

Varicocoele
- Collection of dilated veins in the scrotum due to a problem with the valves.
- Similar to varicose veins in the legs.
- Usually causes no symptoms but can cause discomfort.
- Affects 1 in 7 men.
- Associated with a small increased risk of infertility.

Epididymo-orchitis
- Inflammation of the epididymis and/or testis.
- Commonly caused by an infection (UTI or STI).

Data gathering

Open question
- *"Can you tell me more about your symptoms?"*

Focused/closed questions
HPC: *"Do you have any pain when passing urine, scrotal swelling or discharge from your penis?"*

"Have you noticed any blood in your urine, any weight loss, a testicular lump or pain?" (red flags)

Take a sexual history – see *Appendix 2*.

PMH: Any history of testicular problems or sexually transmitted infections?

FH Any family history of testicular problems?

SH Smoking/alcohol/illicit drug use? Occupation?

ICE: *"Do you have any thoughts as to what might be causing your symptoms?"*

"What were you hoping we might be able to do to help?"

Examination:
- Testicular examination (including trans-illumination with pen torch).
- Examination of lymph nodes.

Clinical management

Investigations
- Scrotal ultrasound scan.
- Urine dipstick and/or MC&S
- STI screening – urethral swab and urine sample.

Management

- Hydrocoele – can leave alone or offer surgery/drainage.
- Varicocoele – can leave alone, or offer surgery to tie off enlarged veins or injection therapy to block affected veins.
- Epididymo-orchitis – antibiotics and/or analgesia. See www.bashh.org/guidelines for further information.
- Safety net – if symptoms not improving to review again.

Role play

Information for doctor	Additional information for role player
Patient: Mr AJ *Age*: 28 years old *SH*: Unemployed, lives alone, single *PMH*: Nil *DH*: Nil *Information*: You are a GP partner and have never seen this patient before.	*PC*: Painful scrotum. *HPC*: 1 week history of scrotal pain. Urethral discharge. **Dysuria. No testicular swelling or masses. Had unprotected sexual intercourse with casual female partner 2 weeks ago.** Not ever had STI check. *ICE*: Worried about an STI. *O/E*: Apyrexial. Tenderness and swelling of epididymis.

Vasectomy

- Male sterilisation.
- Permanent form of contraception.
- Available on NHS but reversal is usually not.

Data gathering

Open question

- *"Can you tell me a bit more about why you would like a vasectomy?"*

Focused/closed questions

HPC: *"Are you currently in a relationship?" "If so, how old is your partner?"*

"Have you had children in the past?" "If so, how many?" "Are these with the same partner?"

"What are you currently using for contraception?"

"Have you discussed the vasectomy with your partner?" "How does she feel?"

PMH: Any medical conditions or previous surgery?

SH: Who lives with you at home? Occupation?

ICE: *"Do you know what a vasectomy entails?"*

Examination:
- BMI.
- Blood pressure.

Clinical management

Explanation to patient
- Small operation to cut the vas deferens (the tube that takes sperm from the testes to the penis).
- If the vas deferens is cut, the sperm are unable to get into the semen that is ejaculated during sex.
- It can be done under local anaesthetic.
- The failure rate is about 1 in 2000.
- You may experience some tenderness and bruising afterwards, but a vasectomy has no effect on sex drive.
- Approximately 8 weeks after the operation you will need to produce two semen samples approx 3–6 weeks apart to ensure that these samples are clear of sperm. You should use contraception with your partner until these semen samples are clear of sperm.
- Offer information leaflet www.nhs.uk/conditions/Vasectomy/Pages/Introduction2.aspx.

Management
- Refer to a urologist for a vasectomy.
- Safety net – GP to review if any further concerns or complications post-operatively.

Role play

Information for doctor	Additional information for role player
Patient: Mr JR *Age*: 40 years old *SH*: Solicitor. Lives with wife, has 3 children. *PMH*: IDDM *DH*: Novorapid, Levemir. *Information*: You are a locum GP. This patient came to see the nurse last week for a routine diabetic check. He mentioned that he wanted a vasectomy.	*PC*: **Has 3 children all with the same partner (aged 42 years).** Has discussed with his wife and they both don't want any more children. **They have been using condoms for contraception.** *ICE*: Wants a permanent method of contraception as doesn't want any more children.

Sexual health

Chlamydia

- Most common sexually transmitted infection in the UK.
- Causes no symptoms in around 70% of females and 50% of males.
- Caused by the bacterium *Chlamydia trachomatis*.

Data gathering

Open question
- *"Can you tell me more about the symptoms you have been experiencing?"*

Focused/closed questions

HPC: Any vaginal discharge (♀) / discharge from your penis (♂) / abdominal pain / burning pain when you pass urine / vaginal bleeding (♀)/ penile pain (♂)?
"Any vaginal bleeding in between periods or any bleeding after sex?" (red flags)
Take sexual history – see *Appendix 2*.

SH: Who lives with you at home? Smoking/alcohol/illicit drug history? Are you currently in a relationship?

ICE: *"Do you have any thoughts as to what might be causing these symptoms?"*
"What concerns do you have about these symptoms?"

Examination:
- Abdominal examination.
- Speculum and vaginal examination (♀).
- External genitalia examination including inguinal lymph nodes (♂).

Clinical management (based on *BASSH*, 2006, *UK National guideline for the management of genital tract infection with* Chlamydia trachomatis)

Investigations
- Endocervical swabs for chlamydia and gonorrhoea (♀).
- Mid-stream urine sample for NAATs (chlamydia and gonorrhoea) (♂).
- Vaginal swab – for bacterial vaginosis and candida (♀).
- Screening for other STIs – e.g. blood test for HIV and syphilis.

Explanation to patient

- Chlamydia infection in women usually affects the cervix and/or womb. In men, it affects the urethra (tube) in the penis.
- If you are infected with chlamydia it is essential that you take treatment even if you do not have any symptoms, because the infection may spread and cause serious complications and you can also still pass on the infection to your sexual partner(s).

Management

- Antibiotics – e.g. cefixime 1 g stat.
- Contact tracing.
- Pregnancy test (♀).
- Offer details of local sexual health clinic for more detailed screening.
- Patient education and information leaflet.
- Safety net – if symptoms don't resolve to return to GP.

Role play

Information for doctor	Additional information for role player
Patient: Ms JJ *Age*: 19 years *SH*: College student *PMH*: Nil *DH*: Nil *Information*: Was seen by GP Partner 8 months ago and was treated for chlamydia infection.	*PC*: *"I've had some vaginal discharge for the past few days"* *HPC*: Had unprotected sexual intercourse 10 days ago with casual partner. **LMP 3 weeks ago. Thin clear coloured discharge. No dysuria. No abdominal pain.** *Sexual history* – Vaginal sex only with male partner. *ICE*: **Worried she may have got chlamydia as the guy she had sex with told her after that he had chlamydia.** *O/E*: Purulent yellow discharge seen on speculum examination.

Pelvic inflammatory disease

- PID is an infection of the female upper genital tract (uterus, fallopian tubes and/or ovaries).
- Most cases are due to ascending infection from the cervix or vagina.
- Commonest infective causes are chlamydia or gonorrhoea.
- Most commonly occurs in the 15–25 year age group.

Data gathering

Open question

- *"Can you tell me more about the symptoms you have been experiencing?"*

Focused/closed questions

HPC: *"Have you been experiencing any abdominal pain?" "Where exactly is the pain?"*

"Do you get any pain during intercourse?"

"Do you notice any bleeding after sex or between periods?" (red flags)

"Do you have any pain when passing urine?"

Any vaginal discharge? Fever?

"When was your last menstrual period?" (always consider ectopic pregnancy)

Take sexual history – see *Appendix 2*

PMH: Any previous sexually transmitted infections?

Any previous pelvic surgery?

SH: Smoking/alcohol/illicit drug history? Who lives with you at home? Occupation?

ICE: *"How have these symptoms been generally affecting you?"*

Examination: • Abdominal examination.

• Vaginal examination – check for cervical motion tenderness and adnexal tenderness.

• Speculum examination.

Clinical management

Investigations
- Endocervical swabs for gonorrhoea and chlamydia NAATs.
- Vaginal swab for other infections.
- Pregnancy test.
- Pelvic ultrasound scan and/or laparoscopy – if recommended by a specialist.

Explanation to patient
- Pelvic inflammatory disease is usually caused by an infection in the womb or around the ovaries which has spread up from the vaginal area.
- It usually causes abdominal pain.
- Antibiotics are usually enough to treat the infection and improve symptoms.
- It is important that it is treated early as it can affect your fertility if symptoms go untreated for a long time. In pregnancy, one complication may be an ectopic pregnancy where the fetus grows outside of the womb.

Management (based on *RCOG, 2008, Green-top guideline 32: Pelvic inflammatory disease*)
- Mild–moderate PID – oral ofloxacin 400 mg twice daily plus oral metronidazole 400 mg twice daily for 14 days.
- If severe symptoms, admit to hospital for IV antibiotics and/or consideration for surgery (salpingectomy).
- Also admit to hospital if a surgical emergency cannot be excluded, for PID in pregnancy, tubo-ovarian abscess, or for poor response to oral treatment.

- Offer contact tracing if chlamydia or gonorrhoea are confirmed.
- Safety net – follow up in 72 hours or sooner if necessary and again after treatment is completed.

Role play

Information for doctor	Additional information for role player
Patient: Ms SR *Age*: 21 years *SH*: University student *PMH*: Nil *DH*: Nil *Information*: You are a GP Registrar and SR is a temporary patient.	*PC*: Abdominal pain *HPC*: Pain in lower abdomen intermittently for the past month. Pain during intercourse also. **No IMB/PCB. Has some vaginal discharge – clear thin discharge, no odour.** No dysuria. **LMP 2 weeks ago.** *Sexual history*: **Has had about 10 different sexual partners in the past 6 months.** Last had sex 1 week ago (unprotected sexual intercourse). *ICE*: Worried about STIs as has never been tested. *O/E*: Afebrile. Tenderness in left iliac fossa. Abdomen soft. Mild left adnexal tenderness. Cervical motion tenderness.

Emergency contraception

- Contraception which is taken after unprotected intercourse to protect against pregnancy.
- The three main types are Levonelle and ulipristal pills and the IUCD.

Data gathering

Open question
- *"Why are you requesting emergency contraception today?"*

Focused/closed questions
HPC: *"When did you have unprotected intercourse?"*
"Have there been any other episodes of unprotected intercourse since your last period?"
"When was your last menstrual period?"
"Any abdominal pain?" (red flag)
"Any vaginal bleeding since your last period?"
"Have you used emergency contraception before?"
"What contraception do you usually use?"
PMH: Any past medical problems? Any previous pregnancies?

SH: Smoking/alcohol/illicit drug history? Relationship? Who lives with you at home? Support? Occupation?

ICE: *"Do you know how emergency contraception works?"*

Examination • Abdominal examination – if there is abdominal pain.

Clinical management

Investigations
- Not required.

Explanation to patient
- Emergency contraception is used to prevent you getting pregnant if you have unprotected sex.
- There are two main types – the emergency contraceptive pill or an IUCD which can be inserted up to five days after having unprotected sex.
- The pill is the most commonly used emergency contraception. The progesterone pill is called Levonelle, and this is taken as a one-off dose as soon as possible after unprotected sex. It either prevents or delays the release of an egg or prevents the fertilised egg from implanting in the womb. If used within 24 hours of unprotected intercourse it is about 95% effective. If used within 48 hours it is 85% effective, and if used within 72 hours it is about 58% effective. If a patient vomits within 2 hours they should take another pill as soon as possible.
- There is a new emergency contraceptive pill, ulipristal, which was found to be 97% effective if used within 72 hours in a recent study (*Faculty of Sexual and Reproductive Healthcare*, 2009, *New product review October*). It is only licensed for women over 18 years.
- The IUCD (copper coil) can be used for emergency contraception (it is the most effective option) and then for on-going contraception.
- If after using emergency contraception your next period is late, it is important that you do a pregnancy test and see your GP as soon as possible.

Management
- Levonelle or ulipristal.
- IUCD.
- Contraception advice and education.
- Sexual health promotion.
- Give patient information leaflet – www.fpa.org.uk.
- Safety net – if next period is delayed or very light come back to see GP.

Role play

Information for doctor	Additional information for role player
Patient: Ms LJ *Age*: 15 years *SH*: School pupil, smokes 10 cigs/day *PMH*: Asthma *DH*: Salbutamol, beclomethasone	*PC*: "*I had unprotected sex 2 days ago and would like the morning after pill*" *HPC*: **Had unprotected sexual intercourse with casual partner 48 hours ago.** Not on any regular contraception. No other episodes of unprotected sexual intercourse since last period. No abdominal pain. No previous pregnancies. **Never had STI check before. LMP 3 weeks ago.** *ICE*: Worried about getting pregnant.

Combined oral contraceptive pill

- Contains two hormones, progesterone and oestrogen.
- Works by preventing ovulation, thickening cervical mucus to prevent fertilisation and thinning the lining of the uterus to prevent implantation.
- It is over 99% effective if used correctly.
- In England, Wales and Northern Ireland it is lawful to provide contraceptive advice and treatment to young people without parental consent, provided that the practitioner is satisfied that the Fraser criteria for competence are met:
  - The young person understands the practitioner's advice.
  - The young person cannot be persuaded to inform their parents, or will not allow the practitioner to inform the parents, that contraceptive advice has been sought.
  - The young person is likely to begin or to continue having intercourse with or without contraceptive treatment.
  - Unless she receives contraceptive advice or treatment, the young person's physical or mental health (or both) are likely to suffer.
- In Scotland, although the Fraser Guidelines are sometimes used by health professionals, they have no authority in Scottish law. The only criterion when determining 'competency' is that the child understands the nature and consequence of the treatment.

Data gathering

Open question
- "*Why would you like to start taking the combined contraceptive pill?*"

Focused/closed questions
HPC: "*When was your last menstrual period?*"
"*Are your periods regular?*"
"*Are you currently using any form of contraception?*"

"Do you suffer with heavy periods?"

"Do you ever suffer from migraines?" "If so, do you experience any warning signs beforehand, e.g. flashing lights?" (red flag)

PMH: Any history of high blood pressure, liver disease, breast cancer or DVT? (red flags)

FH: Any family history of breast cancer, DVT, stroke or heart disease?

DH: Do you take any regular medications? St John's Wort? Enzyme inducers, e.g. carbamazepine, rifampicin?

SH: Do you smoke?

ICE: "What do you know about the pill?"

Examination:
- BP.
- BMI.

Clinical management

Investigations
- Nil

Explanation to patient
- The most common type of pill is the 21 day pill, in which each month you take one tablet a day for 21 days and then no tablets for 7 days. During the 7 day break you will expect to get a 'withdrawal' bleed.
- If you start the pill on the first day of your period, or up to day 5 of a regular 28 day cycle, you will be protected from pregnancy straight away. If you start the pill at any other time, you will need to use additional contraception for the first 7 days after starting the pill.
- The advantages of the combined pill are, it usually makes your bleeds regular, lighter and less painful. It may also help with premenstrual symptoms, and it may reduce the risk of cancer of the ovary, uterus and colon. It may also protect against pelvic inflammatory disease.
- The disadvantages are that you may experience side effects, such as headaches, nausea, breast tenderness and mood changes. The pill may also increase your blood pressure, and it does not protect against sexually transmitted infections. There is also a slight increased risk of developing a DVT. Research suggests that there may be a very small increased risk of developing breast cancer or cervical cancer with longer use of hormonal contraception.
- Missing one pill anywhere in the pack, or starting the pill one day late is not a problem. If you have missed more than one pill, refer to the missed pill rules (www.fpa.org.uk).
- If you take a course of antibiotics whilst on the pill you should use extra precautions while taking the antibiotics and for 7 days afterwards. Similarly if you have diarrhoea the pill may be less effective and extra precautions may be needed.

Management
- Six monthly pill check (including BP check).

- Patient education, including an information leaflet and explanation of the missed pill rules.

Role play

Information for doctor	Additional information for role player
Patient: Ms JE *Age*: 15 years *SH*: Lives with parents. School pupil. Non-smoker *FH*: Nil *PMH*: Nil *Information*: You are a GP registrar.	*PC*: *"I would like to start on the pill"* *HPC*: Has a new boyfriend and they have started being sexually active. **Using condoms currently. LMP 3 weeks ago. No history of DVT/breast cancer/migraine.** *ICE*: Wants to try the pill as some of her friends at school take it. *O/E*: BP 120/80 mmHg, BMI – 23.

Termination of pregnancy

- One-fifth of all pregnancies are terminated worldwide.
- 90% of all abortions are carried out at under 13 weeks of gestation.
- The 1967 Abortion Act allows termination before 24 weeks of gestation if:
    - it reduces the risk to a woman's life, or
    - it reduces the risk to her physical or mental health, or
    - it reduces the risk to the physical or mental health of her existing children, or
    - the baby is at substantial risk of being seriously mentally or physically handicapped.
- There is no upper limit on gestational time if there is a risk to the mother's life or risk of grave permanent injury to the mother's physical/mental health or if there is substantial risk that, if the child were born, it would suffer such physical or mental abnormalities as to be seriously handicapped.

Data gathering

Open question
- *"Why do you want to have a termination?"*

Focused/closed questions
HPC: *"When was your last menstrual period?"*
"Have you ever been pregnant before?"
"Were you using any contraception?" "If so, what?"
"Have you got any abdominal pain or fever?" (red flags)
"Have you thought about other options, for example adoption?"
PMH: *"Have you had any previous terminations?"*

"*Have you had any previous pelvic surgery?*"
Any history of depression?

SH: "*Are you currently in a relationship?*" "*Have you discussed this with your partner?*"
Who lives with you at home? Support network?
Occupation?

ICE: "*Do you have any ideas about what a termination entails?*"
"*Do you have any concerns about having a termination?*"

Examination: • Abdominal examination.

Clinical management

Investigations
- Ultrasound scan – dating and viability scan undertaken prior to the TOP.

Explanation to patient
- There are different types of termination depending on how many weeks pregnant you are:
  - Medical termination (up to 9 weeks pregnant) – you attend a hospital/clinic twice, on two separate days. You are given two medications 48 hours apart (mifepristone and prostaglandin). Mifepristone blocks the hormones that help a pregnancy to continue. Prostaglandins make your womb contract and cause vaginal bleeding and cramping to expel the products of the pregnancy.
  - Vacuum aspiration is used for pregnancies between 7 and 12 weeks of pregnancy. A tube is inserted into your womb through the cervix and suction is applied to remove the womb contents.
  - Dilation and evacuation (D&E) is used for pregnancies between 12 and 19 weeks. It is a surgical procedure whereby the neck of the womb is dilated and the womb is evacuated of its contents.

Management
- Counsel the patient to ensure she is comfortable with her decision.
- Refer for termination of pregnancy, e.g. Marie Stopes Clinic (note that as a doctor, it is your legal right to refuse to certify a woman for an abortion if you have a moral objection, although you should refer immediately to another doctor who is willing to certify the patient).
- Arrange follow-up which should include a discussion about contraception and counselling if required.
- Safety net – see GP or go straight to A&E if fever or abdominal pain.

Role play

Information for doctor	Additional information for role player
Patient: Ms AL *Age*: 25 years *SH*: Waitress, lives with boyfriend *FH*: Nil *PMH*: Nil *DH*: Nil *Information*: Newly registered patient. You are a locum GP.	*PC*: *"'I've just found out that I'm pregnant and I would like to have a termination".* *HPC*: LMP 7 weeks ago. **No previous pregnancies.** Was using condoms but sometimes forgot. Hasn't discussed with boyfriend. Doesn't want to tell him. Not keen on alternative options. No abdominal pain or fever. *SH*: **Has a supportive friend she can talk to.** *ICE*: **Doesn't feel ready to have children yet. Not financially stable. Having relationship problems also.**

Care of people with cancer and palliative care

Palliative care/pain management

- GPs will often be the first point of contact for palliative care patients in the community.
- Common problems encountered in palliative care include inadequate pain control, vomiting, constipation and depression.
- It is important that the patient feels well supported in the community, and GPs should work alongside the community palliative care team, to offer ongoing help and support to the patient and their families.

Data gathering

Open question
- *"Can you tell me what problems you have been experiencing?"*

Focused/closed questions

HPC: *"Are you currently experiencing any pain?"* *"If so, where is the pain?"*
"What type of pain is it?" *"How severe is the pain?"*
"Are you experiencing any nausea or vomiting, or any constipation?"
"Are you passing urine OK?"
"Any breathlessness?" (red flag)
"How is your appetite?"
"How is your mood?"
"Are you sleeping OK?"

DH: *"What medications are you currently taking?"*

SH: Who is living with you at home? Support network? How are you coping? Carers? Finances?

ICE: *"How were you hoping we could help you today?"*
"Do you have any particular worries or concerns about your illness?"

Examination: • Specific to symptoms, e.g. abdominal, respiratory, etc.

Clinical management

Investigations
- If abdominal pain, consider abdominal X-ray.
- If SOB, consider CXR.

Explanation to patient
- Palliative care aims to provide relief from pain and other distressing symptoms, and also offers a support system to help you as the patient, and your loved ones through this difficult time.

Management
Pain management
- Use a pain assessment tool to adequately assess the pain before starting or changing analgesics.
- If pain control is required use the analgesic ladder and regularly review:
  - Step 1 (Mild pain) – use paracetamol +/- NSAIDs.
  - Step 2 (Moderate pain) – use weak opioids such as codeine, dihydrocodeine or tramadol.
  - Step 3 (Moderate–severe pain) – use strong opioids. Morphine is the drug of first choice. Start with 5–10 mg 4 hourly (use lower doses in the elderly or those with renal impairment). Increase in 30–50% increments to achieve pain control.
  - If the morphine dose exceeds 300 mg in 24 hours seek specialist advice.
  - When prescribing opiates also prescribe laxatives and if required, an anti-emetic.
  - For maintenance treatment, you can continue with 4-hourly immediate release morphine or change to 12-hourly modified release morphine.

Symptom control (based on *NHS Scotland*, 2009, *Palliative care guidelines*)
- Anorexia – consider metoclopramide 10 mg TDS or domperidone 10–20 mg TDS before meals. Can also consider prescribing corticosteroids for 1 week. If no benefit, stop.
- Breathlessness – treat any reversible causes (e.g. infection, effusion, PE*). Treatment options include oxygen, nebulised sodium chloride to loosen secretions, bronchodilators and dexamethasone.
  *requires hospital treatment.
- Constipation – clarify cause before starting treatment, e.g. opioids, dehydration, immobility, hypercalcaemia. Encourage good fluid intake. Can try senna, Movicol or co-danthramer in terminally ill patients.
- Delirium – causes include opioid or sedative drugs, drug withdrawal, dehydration, urinary retention or electrolyte disturbance. Treat any underlying causes. First line drug is haloperidol 0.5–3 mg PO or SC daily. Second choice is benzodiazepines, e.g. lorazepam 0.5–1 mg PO or SL. Nurse in quiet area with minimal noise and adequate lighting.

- Nausea and vomiting – seek and treat any reversible causes (e.g. medications, infection, constipation, hypercalcaemia). Treatments include metoclopramide, domperidone and cyclizine.
- Emergencies:
  - Haemorrhage – give sedation if distressed and/or dying patient. Consider emergency referral.
  - Hypercalcaemia – hydration and bisphosphonates.
  - Seizures – prophylactic anticonvulsant if structural cause. Midazolam or rectal diazepam if dying patient.
  - Spinal cord compression – emergency referral to A&E.
- Last days of life – when all reversible causes for the patient's deterioration have been considered, the multi-disciplinary team should agree the patient is dying and change the goals of care. Resuscitation status should be clarified and documented. For further details refer to www.endoflifecare.nhs.uk/eolc or www.mcpcil.org.uk/liverpool_care_pathway.
- Safety net – arrange for regular review and encourage patient to seek advice if symptoms not improving or worsening.

Role play

Information for doctor	Additional information for role player
Patient: Mrs JC *Age*: 47 years *SH*: Married with 2 children. Currently receiving disability living allowance. *PMH*: Metastatic breast cancer. *DH*: Oxycontin 40 mg BD, oxynorm 10 mg QDS, lactulose 10 ml BD. *Information*: Booked emergency appointment today. You are a salaried GP.	*PC*: "*I have a lot of back pain and am having difficulty getting out of the house now*". *HPC*: Worsening back pain for the past couple of days. Pain over vertebrae. No radiation. Has to walk with a stick. Is already taking high doses of analgesia. Bowels last opened 2 days ago. No nausea. Passing urine OK. No leg numbness. *ICE*: Would like some stronger pain relief. *O/E*: Cachectic. Tenderness over lower lumbar vertebrae.

Mental health

Anxiety

- Generalised anxiety disorder is a condition where you have excessive anxiety on most days.
- The cause is unknown, although it may be triggered by a stressful event or there may be a genetic component.
- Treatment includes CBT, medication or self help.

Data gathering

Open question
- *"Can you tell me more about the anxiety you have been experiencing?"*
- *"What do you mean when you say you are anxious?"*

Focused/closed questions

HPC: *"How long have you experienced these feelings for?"*
"Are there any particular triggers?"
"Do you ever have an awareness of your heart beating quickly?"
Any SOB/dry mouth/nausea?
"Do you ever experience episodes of feeling irritable?"
"Do you have problems sleeping?"
"Do you ever avoid certain situations due to fear or anxiety?"
"Have you ever had any thoughts of harming yourself or suicide?" (red flags)

PMH: *"Have you ever had any anxiety or panic attacks in the past?"*
Any past history of depression or psychiatric illness?

DH: Are you on any regular medications?

FH: *"Are you aware of any family history of mental illness or anxiety?"*

SH: Who lives with you at home? Support network? Occupation? Smoking/alcohol / illicit drug history? Daily caffeine intake?

ICE: *"How is this problem affecting your day to day life?"*

Examination: • Blood pressure, pulse.
• Cardiac examination.

Clinical management

Investigations

- ECG

Explanation to patient

- Anxiety is the unpleasant feeling you get when you feel worried, uneasy or distressed about something that may or may not be about to happen.
- It can result in physical symptoms such as nausea, dry mouth, rapid breathing and fast heart rate.
- Feeling anxious is sometimes perfectly normal. However, people with generalised anxiety disorder find it hard to control their worries. Their feelings of anxiety are more constant and often affect their daily life.

Management (based on NICE, 2004, CG22: Anxiety)

- Self help strategies.
- Exercise.
- Cognitive behavioural therapy.
- SSRI.
- Benzodiazepines can be used, but not for longer than 2–4 weeks.
- If no improvement despite the above measures, refer to psychiatry.
- Offer information about support groups.
- Safety net – arrange follow-up appointment to monitor progress.

Role play

Information for doctor	Additional information for role player
Patient: Mr SW *Age*: 43 years *SH*: Single, works as an investment banker, smoker, drinks 40 units alcohol/wk *PMH*: Depression *DH*: Fluoxetine 40 mg OD *FH*: Brother has depression. *Information*: You are a GP Partner. You last saw this patient 1 month ago for a medication review.	*PC*: Feeling very anxious. Has had panic attacks whilst on the train going to work. *HPC*: Difficulty concentrating, **poor sleep**. Has a very stressful job. Generally low mood. Gets dry mouth and palpitations during panic attacks. Also hyperventilates. *ICE*: **Would like some medication to help with his anxiety.** *O/E*: HR – 90 bpm, regular; BP – 130/80 mmHg; cardiac exam – NAD.

Depression

- Describes a state of persistent low mood, severe enough to interfere with everyday life.
- It affects 1 in 5 people at some point in their lives.

- Symptoms include low mood, loss of interest and enjoyment, low energy, feelings of guilt and worthlessness, and changes in appetite and sleep pattern.
- Management includes watchful waiting, self help, talking therapies and anti-depressants.

Data gathering

Open question
- *"Can you tell me about your low mood?"*

Focused/closed questions

HPC: *"When did you first start feeling low in mood?"*
"Did anything trigger it off?"
How is your sleep/concentration/self esteem?
"How would you describe your energy levels?"
"Do you find that you are not able to enjoy things that are usually pleasurable or interesting?"
How are you functioning at work/college/school?
"Have you ever felt so low that you felt like you didn't want to carry on with life?" (red flag) *"If so, had you made any plans?"* *"What stopped you from following through with these plans?"*

PMH: Any previous problems with depression/mental illness? Any past psychiatric admissions? Any previous suicide/self harm attempts? (red flag)

DH: Are you on any regular medications? (beware of the potentially disinhibiting effects of benzodiazepines in someone depressed and suicidal)

FH: Any family history of depression?

SH: Who lives with you at home? Support network? Occupation? Smoking/alcohol/illicit drug history?

Examination: • Mental state examination (see *Appendix 3*).

Clinical management

Investigations
- Nil specific – clinical diagnosis.

Explanation to patient
- The word 'depression' is used to describe everyday feelings of low mood which can affect us all from time to time. Feeling sad or fed up is a normal reaction to experiences that are upsetting, stressful or difficult; those feelings will usually pass.
- If you are affected by depression, you are not 'just' sad or upset. You have an illness which means that intense feelings of persistent sadness, helplessness and hopelessness are accompanied by physical effects such as sleeplessness and loss of energy.

Management (based on *NICE, 2009, CG90: Depression in adults (update)*)

- Give patient a PHQ-9 questionnaire to complete.
- Exercise.
- If mild depression, consider watchful waiting or recommend a guided self help programme based on CBT.
- In mild to moderate depression, consider short term psychological treatment (e.g. CBT or counselling).
- In severe depression consider combination treatment of an anti-depressant (SSRI) and individual CBT.
- If immediate risk to self or others, consider an urgent referral to the mental health services.
- Safety net – always arrange follow-up and ask the patient to return sooner if their depressive symptoms worsen.

Role play

Information for doctor	Additional information for role player
Patient: Mr HA *Age*: 34 years *SH*: Unemployed. Lives alone. Wife in Pakistan with his children. *FH*: Nil *PMH*: Back pain *DH*: Tramadol, Nurofen *Information*: Last consultation for back pain 1 week ago with locum GP. You are a salaried GP.	*PC*: "*I'm having trouble sleeping*". *HPC*: Has difficulty getting to sleep and then wakes up several times in the night. **Feels low in mood.** Rarely leaves the house now. No energy. **Some suicidal thoughts but no plans and his family would prevent him from doing this.** Poor concentration. *ICE*: **Thinks low mood could be due to loneliness and also constant back pain.** *O/E*: Mental state examination – objectively and subjectively low mood.

Sleep disorders

- Up to 30% of the adult population have been affected by sleep problems at some time, especially the elderly.
- Problems include getting to sleep, staying asleep, waking too early, or disturbed sleep.
- Sleep problems can occur for various different reasons – medical reasons, emotional reasons, unhelpful surroundings or disturbed sleep routines.

Data gathering

Open question
- "*What problems have you been experiencing with your sleep?*"

Focused/closed questions

HPC: *"When did these problems first start?"*

"Are you aware of any particular triggers?"

"Do you have problems getting to sleep, staying asleep or waking too early?"

"Has your usual sleep routine or environment changed recently?"

"How is your general mood?"

PMH: Any history of depression or psychiatric problems?

Any medical conditions?

DH: Do you take any regular medications, e.g. stimulant medication?

"Have you tried any medication for your sleeping problem?"

SH: Who lives with you at home? Any relationship problems?

Occupation? Stress at work? Smoking/alcohol/illicit drug history? Caffeine intake?

ICE: *"How is this sleep problem impacting on your daily life?"*

Examination: • Nil specific.

Clinical management

Investigations
• Sleep diary and sleep studies.

Management
• Avoid caffeine, alcohol and smoking in the evening.
• Ensure surroundings are amenable to sleep.
• Relaxation, e.g. bath before bedtime.
• Medications, e.g. anti-depressant if related to depression/anxiety (remember that sleeping tablets, for example, diazepam and zopiclone are addictive and ideally should not be given on a regular basis).

Role play

Information for doctor	Additional information for role player
Patient: Mrs EE *Age:* 76 years *SH:* Lives in a residential home. Retired. Non-smoker. No alcohol. *PMH:* Polymyalgia rheumatica *DH:* Prednisolone 5 mg daily. *Information:* Patient contacted the practice this morning requesting a home visit due to problems sleeping. You are a GP Registrar and have agreed to call her to find out further information.	*PC:* *"I'm having terrible trouble sleeping doctor".* *HPC:* Difficulty getting to sleep and also wakes up several times in the night. Feels very sleepy during the day. **Mood fine. Drinks a lot of tea including before bedtime. Goes to the toilet 2–3 times each night.** *ICE:* Would like some sleeping tablets.

Deliberate self harm

- DSH describes acts such as self cutting or self poisoning, in which a patient deliberately causes harm or injury to themself, with or without suicidal intent.
- Self harm is most common in adolescence and early adulthood, and in those with psychiatric or personality disorders.
- Treatment includes psychological therapies and anti-depressant medications.

Data gathering

Open questions
- *"Can you tell me why you deliberately tried to harm yourself?"*
- *"Can you tell me more about what happened?"*

Focused/closed questions

HPC: *"What was your reason for deliberately trying to harm yourself?"*
"Had you been planning this beforehand?" (red flag)
"Did you write a suicide note beforehand?" (red flag)
"Did you plan it so that you wouldn't be found?" (red flag)
"How did you feel whilst you were harming yourself?"
"How do you feel about it now? What is stopping you from harming yourself now?"
"Was it more of a cry for help or did you seriously want to end your life?"

PMH: *"Have you ever tried to deliberately harm yourself before or have you ever tried to take your own life before?"* (red flag) Any past history of depression?

FH: Any family history of mental health problems or deliberate self harming?

DH: Do you currently take any regular medications? Anti-depressants? Anti-psychotics?

SH: Who lives with you at home? Occupation/School/College? Support network? Alcohol/smoking/illicit drug history?

ICE: *"What help would you like to prevent you from deliberately harming yourself again?"*
"How has your self harming affected your relationship with your family?"

Examination:
- Mental state examination (see *Appendix 3*).
- Physical examination relevant to specific self injury.

Clinical management

Investigations

- Risk assessment (consider red flags, e.g. psychiatric illness, suicidal intent, poor social support, drug abuse, risk of harm to self and others).

Explanation to patient

- There are many different reasons why people deliberately self harm, for example, to find relief from a terrible situation or as a way of coping with their emotions or feelings.
- There are a number of different methods that can be used to treat self harm and which concentrate on either treating the underlying causes or on treating the behaviour itself.

Management (NICE, 2004, CG16: Self-harm)

- Urgently establish physical risk and mental state.
- Always offer physical treatment.
- Refer to A&E urgently if the patient is at significant risk of self injury.
- Support groups.
- Self-help guide (www.ntw.nhs.uk/pic/leaflets/Self%20Harm.pdf).
- Consider referral for psychological therapy.
- Consider anti-depressants if history of depression.
- Be vigilant when prescribing drugs to people who have previously self poisoned.
- Safety net – review again within the next week.

Role play

Information for doctor	Additional information for role player
Patient: Ms SW *Age*: 18 years *SH*: Lives with parents. College student. Smokes 10 cigs/day and also smokes cannabis. Drinks 30 units alcohol/week. *PMH*: Depression, self harm *DH*: Fluoxetine 20 mg daily *Information*: Was reviewed yesterday by the mental health crisis team after an episode of self harm. You are a GP Registrar.	*PC*: "*My mum wanted me to come to see you today because I self harmed yesterday*" *HPC*: "*I cut my wrists and arms*". **Superficial cuts. Felt fed up. Feels low. Parents were at home downstairs at the time.** No suicidal intent. Feels silly about it now. Didn't plan it beforehand. *FH*: No family history of mental illness. *ICE*: Willing to have some talking therapy.

Cardiovascular

Angina pectoris

- Clinical syndrome characterised by discomfort usually in the chest, arm or jaw, precipitated by activities such as exercise which increase myocardial oxygen demand.
- Usually caused by coronary atherosclerosis, resulting in ischaemia of the heart vessels.
- Angina can be classified as stable or unstable:
  - Stable angina refers to a sensation of discomfort or pain in the chest, arm or jaw brought on by exertion, and relieved by rest or GTN.
  - Unstable angina is characterised by episodes of chest pain at rest, or increasingly rapidly with exertion, and which increase in frequency or severity. There is no ST elevation seen on an ECG.
- Risk factors for angina include hypertension, hypercholesterolaemia, smoking, physical inactivity and being overweight.

Data gathering

Open question

- *"Can you describe the chest pain that you have been experiencing?"*

Focused/closed questions

HPC: *"Where do you feel the pain?"*
"Does the pain spread anywhere else?"
"How would you describe the pain?"
"How severe is the pain on a scale of 1 to 10?"
"Does anything make the pain better or worse?"
"Do you have any associated shortness of breath?"
"Do you wake up at night short of breath?" "How many pillows do you need to sleep with?"
"Have you noticed any nausea, clamminess or sensation that your heart is pounding?" (red flags)

PMH: Any previous heart problems or surgery?

DH: Do you take any regular medications?

FH: Any family history of heart problems?

SH: Smoking/alcohol/illicit drug history? Occupation?

ICE: *"What do you think might be causing the chest pain?"*

Examination:
- BP, pulse.
- Cardiovascular system.

Clinical management

Investigations
- Blood test – FBC, U&Es, TFTs, LFTs, fasting glucose and cholesterol.
- ECG.
- Exercise test (or alternatively myocardial perfusion scintigraphy).
- Coronary angiogram – if high risk or unclear diagnosis.

Explanation to patient
- Angina describes the pain caused by narrowing of the heart arteries. There is a reduced blood supply to parts of the heart muscle.
- This blood supply may be enough to supply the heart when you are resting, but if you exert yourself the heart may not have enough blood and oxygen to function adequately.

Management (based on *SIGN*, 2007, *96: Management of stable angina* and *NICE*, 2010, *CG95: Chest pain of recent onset*)
- If unstable angina, give 300 mg aspirin and immediate referral to hospital.
- Otherwise refer to the chest pain clinic for confirmation of the diagnosis and to assess the severity.
- Lifestyle modifications – stop smoking, treat high blood pressure, healthy diet, weight loss and exercise, reduce alcohol intake.
- Glyceryl trinitrate (GTN) used as required when the angina pain develops – relaxes the blood vessels reducing the load on the heart.
- Aspirin 75 mg daily and long term statin.
- Beta-blockers – first line drug, reduces the rate and force of the heart beat (if intolerant, alternatives include calcium channel blockers, long acting nitrates and nicorandil).
- Calcium channel blockers – second line.
- Refer to cardiology if symptoms not controlled despite maximum therapeutic doses of two drugs.
- ACE inhibitor – in patients with reduced LVF or with a past history of MI.
- Immunisations – pneumococcus and annual influenza.
- Inform DVLA (cannot hold an HGV licence).

Role play

Information for doctor	Additional information for role player
Patient: Mr MK *Age*: 63 years *SH*: Lives with wife. Retired *PMH*: Diabetes, hypertension *DH*: Ramipril 5 mg OD, metformin 850 mg TDS, gliclazide 80 mg OD *Information*: Saw nurse yesterday for BP check – 150/95 mmHg. You are a locum GP.	*PC*: *"I have been getting some chest pain".* *HPC*: Chest pain only on exertion. Pain in centre of chest with some radiation into the neck. **Pain lasts 1–2 mins each time. Rest relieves the pain. No palpitations, nausea or clamminess. Slight SOB with the pain.** *ICE*: Worried about his heart because is diabetic and has high blood pressure *O/E*: CVS exam – NAD.

Peripheral vascular disease

- Disease of the arteries whereby the arteries become narrowed, restricting blood flow to the muscles of the limbs. This can result in intermittent claudication.
- A common symptom is calf pain brought on by exercise and relieved by rest.
- Risk factors include smoking, obesity, inactivity, hypertension, diabetes and high cholesterol.

Data gathering

Open question
- *"Can you describe the pain in the calf that you've been experiencing?"*

Focused/closed questions
HPC: *"When did the problem first start?"*
"Do you experience the pain at rest?" (red flag)
"How far can you walk before the onset of the pain?"
"Have you experienced any cramping of the legs?"
"Are both legs affected?"
"Have you noticed any colour changes in the foot?" (red flag)
"Have you noticed any swelling of your calves?" (red flag)
PMH: Any past history of heart disease? Any history of high blood pressure, high cholesterol or diabetes?
DH: Are you on any regular medications?
FH: Any family history of heart disease or diabetes?
SH: Smoking/alcohol/illicit drug history? Occupation? Stairs at home?
ICE: *"Does this problem stop you from doing things that you would normally be able to do?"*

Examination: • BP, pulse.
• Cardiovascular system.
• Examination of leg – temperature, colour, peripheral pulses.

Clinical management

Investigations
• Routine bloods – FBC, U&Es, fasting lipids and glucose.
• ECG.
• Ankle brachial pressure index.
• Doppler ultrasound scan.

Explanation to patient
• This is a narrowing of one or more arteries, and it mainly affects the arteries that supply blood to the legs. It is due to fatty plaques developing on the inside lining of the blood vessels.

Management
• Smoking cessation, exercise, weight loss, reduce alcohol intake.
• Consider use of aspirin and statins.
• Treat any identifiable causes, e.g. hypertension, diabetes.
• Safety net – return if symptoms not improving or getting worse.
• Refer to vascular surgery urgently if rest pain, absent foot pulses, pallor or evidence of gangrene.

Role play

Information for doctor	Additional information for role player
Patient: Mr SA *Age:* 58 years *SH:* Lives alone. Widowed. Restaurant owner. Ex-smoker (20 pack years), no alcohol. *FH:* Nil *PMH:* MI 2004 *DH:* Aspirin 75 mg daily, simvastatin 40 mg daily. *Information:* You are a salaried GP.	*PC:* Calf pain. *HPC:* 3 week history of bilateral calf pain brought on by exertion and relieved by rest. **Pain brought on after 200 m walking. No SOB or chest pain. No swelling of the calves.** No oedema. No colour changes in the foot or lower leg. *ICE:* Would like to know what is causing the pain. Unable to go out much due to this pain. *O/E:* CVS exam – NAD. Calves soft, non-tender. No calf swelling bilaterally.

Palpitations

- Awareness of your own heartbeat.
- Can be caused by cardiac problems, for example, atrial fibrillation, or from anxiety.
- Requires urgent referral if suspected or proven ventricular tachycardia.

Data gathering

Open question
- *"Can you describe in more detail the palpitations you have been experiencing?"*

Focused/closed questions

HPC: *"When did you first start being aware of your own heartbeat?"*
"How frequently is this occurring?"
"Do you feel your heart beating regularly or irregularly?"
"Could you tap out the rhythm of your heartbeat on the table?"
"Have you noticed any associated shortness of breath or chest pain?"
(red flags)
"Do you have any episodes of dizziness, clamminess or collapse?"
(red flags)
"How much caffeine do you drink on a daily basis?"
"Have you been feeling more anxious than usual?"
"Do you have a fever?"
"Have you been feeling more tired than usual?"
"Any changes to your weight?"

PMH: Any history of anxiety or previous heart problems?

DH: Do you take any regular medications, e.g. bronchodilators, amlodipine or levothyroxine? Have you been taking any cold decongestants?

FH: Any family history of heart problems, thyroid problems, anxiety or unexplained death?

SH: Alcohol/smoking/illicit drug history? Cocaine/amphetamines?

ICE: *"What particularly concerned you about these palpitations?"*

Examination:
- BP, pulse.
- Check for anaemia.
- CVS examination.
- Thyroid examination – if any other symptoms.

Clinical management

Investigations
- 12-lead ECG.

- 24 hour ECG.
- Blood test – FBC, U&Es and TFTs.

Explanation to patient
- Unpleasant awareness of your heartbeat, often described as thumping in your chest.

Management
- Arrange emergency admission for anyone with palpitations with VT or SVT or if additional symptoms of chest pain, SOB or syncope.
- If sinus tachycardia +/- ectopic beats with no adverse features, e.g. structural heart disease, reassure and advise on lifestyle, caffeine and alcohol. If any adverse features, refer to secondary care.
- If AF (chronic or paroxysmal) – refer to NICE guidelines (2006, *CG36: Atrial fibrillation*).
- If related to anxiety, advise self help measures.
- Safety net – if palpitations not resolving, return to the GP.

Role play

Information for doctors	Additional information for role player
Patient: Mr JB *Age*: 24 years *SH*: University student, lives in shared flat *PMH*: Depression *DH*: Fluoxetine 20 mg OD *Information*: Last saw GP 1 week ago for medication review. You are a locum GP.	*PC*: Palpitations. *HPC*: Started experiencing palpitations intermittently since last week. **Fast heart beat but seems regular. Slight SOB also.** No chest pain. Has been under stress recently with university exams. No dizziness. Currently drinks 5–6 cups of coffee each day. Smokes 10 cigs/day. *ICE*: **Worried about his heart.** *O/E*: BP 110/60 mmHg, CV and respiratory exam – NAD.

Respiratory

Asthma

- Common condition affecting the airways of the lungs, resulting in typical symptoms of wheeze, cough, chest tightness and shortness of breath.
- Treatment is usually with inhalers – typically a bronchodilator and/or corticosteroids.

Data gathering

Open question

- *"Can you tell me more about the problems with your breathing?"*

Focused/closed questions

HPC: *"How long have you been experiencing these symptoms for?"*
"Does anything make your breathing better or worse, e.g. cold weather, certain medications or exercise?"
"Do you have a cough, wheeze, shortness of breath, or chest tightness?"
"Is the cough or wheeze worse at any particular time of the day?"
"How regularly do you use your inhalers?" (red flag if uncontrolled symptoms)
"Do you know how to use your inhalers correctly?"
"Have you required any oral steroids in the past year due to breathing problems?" "If so, how many?"

PMH: Any past history of breathing problems? Any previous asthma attacks or hospital admissions due to asthma?

FH: Any family history of asthma, eczema or hayfever?

DH: What medications are you currently taking, e.g. inhalers?

SH: Smoking history? Occupation? Any damp or dust in your home?

ICE: *"What were you hoping we could do to help with this breathing problem?"*
"How does this problem affect you at home/school/work?"

Examination: • Respiratory examination (red flag if respiratory distress or silent chest).
• Peak flow.

Clinical management

Investigations
- Spirometry.
- Reversibility testing.
- CXR – if unclear diagnosis.

Explanation to patient
- A condition affecting the airways of the lungs. The muscles around the walls of the airway tighten so that the airway becomes narrower. The lining of the airways also becomes inflamed and this makes it difficult to breathe, resulting in the symptoms of asthma.

Management (based on *BTS/ SIGN*, 2009, *British guideline on the management of asthma*)
- Lifestyle measures – weight loss, smoking cessation, allergen avoidance.
- Provide a personal written action plan as part of self management education.
- If high probability of asthma, trial of asthma treatment.
- Stepwise management in adults (see BTS guidelines for management of childhood asthma: www.sign.ac.uk/pdf/qrg101.pdf)
  1. Inhaled short-acting beta agonist e.g. salbutamol.
  2. Add inhaled steroid 200–800 mcg/day.
  3. Add inhaled long-acting beta agonist (LABA), e.g. salmeterol. If good response to LABA but control still inadequate, increase the inhaled steroid. If no response to LABA stop this and increase the inhaled steroid.
  4. Add leucotriene receptor antagonist or SR theophylline.
  5. Use daily steroid tablet.
- Admit patients immediately with any features of life threatening asthma or severe asthma not responding to initial treatment.
- Safety net – arrange follow-up to review progress, based on severity of symptoms.

Role play

Information for doctor	Additional information for role player
Patient: Mr JA *Age*: 19 years *SH*: College student, lives with parents *FH*: Asthma, eczema *PMH*: Asthma. No previous hospital admissions *DH*: Salbutamol 1–2 puffs PRN, beclomethasone 2 puffs BD *Information*: Asthma review with nurse 1 week ago – peak flow 250 l/min. You are a salaried GP.	*PC*: Worsening symptoms of asthma, requiring salbutamol several times a day. *HPC*: **Waking at night with cough and chest tightness.** Unable to participate in sports due to breathing problems. Wheeze also. *ICE*: Concerned about not being able to participate in sports as was previously very active and enjoys sports. *O/E*: Chest – bilateral equal air entry. Generalised wheeze throughout both lung fields. Poor inhaler technique.

Chronic obstructive pulmonary disease

- COPD (otherwise referred to as emphysema or bronchitis) is characterised by airflow obstruction which is usually progressive and not fully reversible.
- With emphysema the air sacs of the lungs are gradually destroyed, resulting in difficulty absorbing enough oxygen.
- With chronic bronchitis the airways become narrower, and there is increased mucus production and inflammation.
- A diagnosis of COPD should be considered in those aged over 35 years who are smokers or ex-smokers and who have exertional breathlessness, chronic cough, wheeze or regular sputum production.

Data gathering

Open question
- *"Can you tell me more about your breathing problems?"*

Focused/closed questions
HPC: *"Do you have a cough, wheeze or any shortness of breath?"*
"Have you been coughing up any phlegm?" "If so, what colour is it?"
"Have you noticed any weight loss or blood when you cough?"
(red flag)
"Do you have any chest pain?" (red flag)
"Do you have any ankle swelling or do you wake at night short of breath?" (red flag)

"How frequently do you suffer with chest infections?"

PMH: Any previous chest problems? Any previous hospital admissions due to chest problems?

DH: Regular medications? Inhalers?

FH: Any FH of chest problems?

SH: Smoking history? Occupation? Who lives with you at home? How do you manage at home?

ICE: *"How is your breathing affecting your daily activities?"*

Examination:
- BMI.
- Respiratory examination.
- Peak flow.

Clinical management

Investigation
- CXR – to exclude other causes.
- Spirometry (COPD is defined as FEV_1 <80% and FEV_1/FVC <0.7).
- Determine severity of airflow obstruction (mild COPD = FEV_1 50–80%, moderate COPD = FEV_1 30–49%, severe COPD = FEV_1 <30%).
- FBC (to identify anaemia or polycythaemia).

Explanation to patient
- COPD describes irreversible airway obstruction often caused by smoking.

Management (based on *NICE*, 2010, *CG101: Chronic obstructive pulmonary disease* (*update*))
- Lifestyle measures – smoking cessation, weight loss, exercise.
- Stepwise management:
  1. Short-acting beta agonist, e.g. salbutamol, or antimuscarinic inhaler, e.g. ipratropium.
  2. Add long-acting beta agonist, e.g. salmeterol, or long-acting anticholinergics, e.g. tiotropium (combine these with inhaled corticosteroids if FEV_1 <50%).
  3. Add long-acting muscarinic agonist to the above drugs.
  4. Trial of theophylline.
- Mucolytic drugs – if chronic productive cough.
- Refer to specialist if diagnostic uncertainty, suspected severe COPD, rapid decline in FEV_1, frequent infections or for consideration of long term oxygen therapy.
- Consider long term oxygen therapy if FEV_1 <30%.
- Review people with mild–moderate COPD at least once a year and those with severe COPD at least twice yearly.
- Offer pneumococcal and annual influenza vaccinations.
- Treatment of exacerbations:
  - Increase frequency of bronchodilators and give oral antibiotic if purulent sputum or clinical signs of infection.

- ○ Offer prednisolone 30 mg daily for 7–14 days.
- ○ Safety net – arrange to review and inform patient what to do if symptoms worsen.

Role play

Information for doctor	Additional information for role player
Patient: Mr RM *Age*: 52 years *SH*: Lives with wife. Unemployed. Ex-smoker (20 pack years). *FH*: Nil *PMH*: COPD *DH*: Ipratropium 500 mcg QDS and tiotropium 5 mcg OD. *Information*: Had annual COPD review with nurse yesterday: FEV_1 – 48% FEV_1/FVC – 0.5. You are a GP Partner.	*PC*: "*I feel more breathless even though I'm taking my inhalers regularly*". *HPC*: SOB even with minimal exertion (walking a few yards). Cough with clear sputum production. No recent weight loss. No chest pain. No haemoptysis. Last chest infection 6 months ago. *ICE*: Worried about worsening COPD. *O/E*: Bilateral equal air entry. Widespread wheeze bilaterally.

Gastrointestinal/renal

Dyspepsia

- Symptoms related to problems with digestion.
- Common symptoms include epigastric pain, bloating, nausea or vomiting.
- Causes include 'functional' dyspepsia, duodenal and gastric ulcers, oesophagitis, gastritis, gastro-oesophageal reflux and *Helicobacter pylori* infection.
- Management includes avoidance of triggers, antacids or acid suppressing medication.

Data gathering

Open question
- *"Can you tell me more about these symptoms?"*

Focused/closed questions
HPC: *"Any abdominal pain/nausea/bloating/vomiting?"*
"When did the problem first start?"
"How often do you experience these symptoms?"
"Do you know what triggers the symptoms?"
"Is the problem worse at night or after eating?"
"Any bleeding from the back passage, vomiting blood or weight loss?"
(red flags)
PMH: Any previous stomach problems? Any previous *H. pylori* infection?
FH Any family history of stomach problems?
DH: Do you take any regular medications? NSAIDs/calcium antagonists/bisphosphonates?
SH: Occupation? Stress? Smoking/alcohol/illicit drug history?
ICE: *"Do you have any thoughts as to what is causing these symptoms?"*
Examination: • Abdominal examination.

Clinical management

Investigations
- Bloods – FBC, ferritin.
- *H. pylori* test (either stool antigen, carbon-13 urea breath test or lab-based serology).
- Referral for endoscopy in resistant cases.

Explanation to patient

- Dyspepsia (or indigestion) describes the symptoms that occur when there is a problem with the digestion in the upper gut. Abdominal pain and bloating are common symptoms, and it may be caused by certain medications, for example anti-inflammatory drugs, or by eating certain types of food, for example spicy foods.

Management

- Conservative management – stop smoking, weight loss, avoidance of spicy foods and alcohol.
- Antacids (e.g. Gaviscon) – neutralises stomach acid.
- Stop or change any medications thought to be triggering symptoms.
- If *H. pylori* positive – eradication therapy (refer to *NICE*, 2004, *CG17: Dyspepsia*).
- Acid suppressing medication, e.g. proton pump inhibitors (omeprazole/lansoprazole) or H_2 receptor blockers.
- NICE guidelines (2004, *CG17: Dyspepsia*) – in patients aged 55 years or older with unexplained and persistent recent-onset dyspepsia alone, an urgent referral for endoscopy should be made.
- Safety net – review in 6 weeks if symptoms not improving, or sooner if there is a deterioration in symptoms.

Role play

Information for doctor	Additional information for role player
Patient: Mr TP *Age*: 54 years *SH*: Lives with wife. Taxi driver. Smokes 20 cigs/day. Drinks 50 units alcohol/week. *PMH*: Hypercholesterolaemia *DH*: Simvastatin 40 mg nocte *Information*: You are a GP Registrar.	*PC*: *"I've been getting terrible indigestion, and Gaviscon isn't helping"* *HPC*: Pain in upper abdomen sometimes spreading into the chest. Started 3 weeks ago. **Worse at night and after eating. Some bloating. No obvious food triggers. No vomiting, haemoptysis, melaena or weight loss.** *ICE*: Would like some stronger medication as his friend has a similar problem and was given something from his doctor. *O/E*: Soft abdomen. Mild epigastric tenderness. No palpable masses or organomegaly.

Rectal bleeding

- Refers to gastrointestinal tract bleeding.
- Causes include haemorrhoids, anal fissures, diverticular disease, inflammatory bowel disease or bowel cancer.
- A colonoscopy may be recommended to confirm the diagnosis.

Data gathering

Open question
- *"Can you tell me more about the bleeding from your back passage?"*

Focused/closed questions

HPC: *"When did the bleeding from your back passage start?"*
"Is the blood mixed in with the stool or on the toilet paper?"
"Is the blood bright red or is it darker?"
"Have you noticed any weight loss?" (red flag)
"Any change in bowel habit?" (red flag)
"Any itchiness or soreness around the back passage?"
"Have you passed any mucus in the stools?"
"Are you aware of any abdominal pain?"
"Do you have any pain around your back passage?"
"Have you noticed any dizziness or fatigue?"

PMH: *"Have you had any previous bowel problems or episodes of rectal bleeding?"*

DH: Do you take any regular medications, e.g. warfarin or NSAIDs?

FH: Any family history of bowel problems or bowel cancer?

SH: Smoking/alcohol/illicit drug history?

ICE: *"Do you have any concerns about what might be causing the rectal bleeding?"*

Examination:
- BP and pulse.
- Gastrointestinal examination including digital rectal examination.

Clinical management

Investigations
- Blood test – FBC, ferritin, U&Es, CRP, LFTs, clotting studies.
- Faecal occult blood test.
- Colonoscopy or sigmoidoscopy.

Explanation to patient
- Blood appearing from the back passage.
- Most episodes of rectal bleeding are mild and stop on their own.

Management
- Determined by the diagnosis.
- If any signs of shock, refer to A&E immediately.
- Refer for suspected cancer under the two week wait if:
  - Rectal bleeding plus change of bowel habit persisting for 6 weeks and the patient is 40 years or older.
  - Palpable rectal or right-sided lower abdominal mass.
  - Iron deficiency anaemia without any obvious cause (<11 g/dl in men and <10 g/dl in postmenopausal women).
  - Aged over 60 with rectal bleeding without anal symptoms persisting for 6 weeks.
  - Aged over 60 with change in bowel habit persisting for 6 weeks without rectal bleeding.
- Safety net – if symptoms not improving return to GP.

Role play

Information for doctor	Additional information for role player
Patient: Mr OM *Age*: 34 years *SH*: Lives alone. University lecturer *FH*: Father and paternal grandmother – diabetes. *PMH*: Nil *DH*: Nil *Information*: No previous consultations. You are a GP Partner.	*PC*: "I've been passing blood when I go to the toilet". *HPC*: Six week history of diarrhoea with fresh blood in the stools. **Approx 5 kg weight loss. Also lower abdominal pain when opening bowels. Bowels opening approx 3 times daily.** Fatigue. *ICE*: Very worried about cancer. Has been putting off coming to the doctor. *O/E*: Pallor; abdomen tender in LIF. No palpable masses. Rectal examination – fresh blood, no masses.

Anaemia

- Fewer red blood cells than normal or less haemoglobin than normal in each red blood cell.
- This results in a reduced amount of oxygen being carried around in the blood stream.
- Symptoms include tiredness, lethargy, dizziness, SOB, and headaches.
- Causes include iron deficiency anaemia, haemoglobinopathies, anaemia of chronic disease and B_{12} deficiency.

Data gathering

Open question
- *"Can you tell me what symptoms you have been experiencing?"*

Focused/closed questions

HPC: *"Are you aware of any tiredness, dizziness, breathlessness or headache?"*
"Have you noticed any change in your appetite?"
"Have you felt a sensation of your heart pounding?"
"Has anyone commented that you look paler than usual?"
"Are your periods heavier than usual?"
"Have you noticed any blood in the stools or in the urine?" (red flags)
"Have you noticed any change to your bowel habit or weight loss?" (red flags)
"Do you have a well balanced diet with a variety of meats and vegetables?"
"Have you noticed any bruising or bone pains?" (red flags)

PMH: Any other medical conditions?

DH: Do you take any regular medications, e.g. warfarin, NSAIDs?

SH: Smoking/alcohol/illicit drug history? Occupation? Who lives with you at home?

FH: Any family history of anaemia or any blood disorders?

ICE: "What do you think is causing your anaemia?"

Examination:
- Check for conjunctival pallor, gum hypertrophy, and koilonychia.
- Pulse, BP.
- Cardiovascular system – check for systolic ejection murmur.
- Abdominal examination – if suspected GI cause.

Clinical management

Investigations

- Blood tests – FBC, ferritin, B_{12}, folate, blood film, haemoglobin electrophoresis.
- Faecal occult blood – to determine if any GI blood loss.
- Endoscopy or colonoscopy – to determine site of blood loss.

Explanation to patient

- Red blood cells carry oxygen around the body in a substance called haemoglobin. Haemoglobin gives your blood its red colour. Iron is an important part of haemoglobin.
- If you don't have enough red blood cells, or enough of the oxygen-carrying substance haemoglobin, you have anaemia.
- Anaemia can result from an increased loss or rate of destruction of red blood cells or decreased production of red blood cells.

Management (based on *NHS CKS*, 2008, *Anaemia – iron deficiency – management*)

- Address underlying cause, e.g. menorrhagia, stopping NSAIDs.
- Increase dietary intake of iron (red meat, green vegetables, pulses), vitamin B_{12} (meat, milk, cheese, eggs) and folate (liver, yeast extract, green leafy vegetables).

- Vitamin supplements.
- Ferrous sulphate 200 mg two to three times daily – if iron deficiency anaemia (recheck FBC after 2–4 weeks to assess response to treatment).
- Vitamin B_{12} injections – if vitamin B_{12} deficient (refer urgently to specialist if any neurological involvement or if pregnant).
- Refer to specialist if unexplained iron deficiency anaemia.
- Refer for blood transfusion if Hb <9 and symptomatic.
- Safety net – return to GP if symptoms no better after 2–4 weeks.

Role play

Information for doctor	Additional information for role player
Patient: Ms BN *Age*: 25 years *SH*: Lives with boyfriend and 18 month old baby. Hairdresser. *PMH*: Nil *DH*: Nil *Information*: Last consultation with GP for IUCD insertion 6 months ago. You are a salaried GP.	*PC*: "*My boyfriend thinks I look paler than usual, so I wanted to check if I'm anaemic*". *HPC*: Feels more tired than usual. **Periods have been heavier.** No SOB. No dizziness or headache. No weight loss. Had anaemia in pregnancy. **Vegetarian.** *ICE*: Having difficulty going to work due to tiredness and low energy levels. *O/E*: Pallor. Heart rate regular. Abdominal examination – NAD.

Irritable bowel syndrome

- IBS is a common disorder affecting the digestive system due to a problem with the function of the gut.
- Symptoms include abdominal pain, diarrhoea, constipation and bloating.
- Approximately 10–20% of people will be affected by IBS at any one time in the UK (*NICE, 2008, CG61: Irritable bowel syndrome*).
- Treatment includes dietary advice, antispasmodic medication, constipation medication or psychological therapy.

Data gathering

Open question
- "*Can you tell me about the bowel symptoms you have been experiencing?*"

Focused/closed questions
HPC: "*Do you have any abdominal pain or bloating?*"
         "*Where exactly is the abdominal pain?*"
         "*How long have you had these symptoms for?*"
         "*Is the abdominal pain relieved by opening your bowels?*"

> *"Have you noticed a change in your bowel habit, weight loss or bleeding from your back passage?"* (red flags)
>
> *"Have you passed any mucus in your stools?"*

PMH: Any previous history of bowel problems? Any previous operations on your bowel?

FH: Any FH of bowel problems?

DH: Are you taking any regular medications?

SH: Smoking/alcohol history? Occupation?

ICE: *"Do you have any particular concerns about your bowel problems?"*

Examination:
- Abdominal examination.

Clinical management

Investigations
- Blood test (FBC, ESR, CRP, endomysial antibodies (EMA) or tissue transglutaminase (TTG) for coeliac disease).
- Colonoscopy – if need to rule out bowel cancer.

Explanation to patient
- IBS is a condition affecting the function of the gut. It is thought that there may be over-activity of part of the bowel.

Management (based on *NICE*, 2008, *CG61: Irritable bowel syndrome*)
- Reassurance – does not lead to bowel cancer.
- Symptom diary.
- Regular meals and at least 8 glasses of water/fluid daily.
- Restrict tea/coffee/fizzy drinks/alcohol.
- Limit fresh fruit and high fibre food.
- Probiotics – some evidence suggests these can help.
- Regular exercise.
- Medications – e.g. buscopan, lactulose, loperamide, tricyclic anti-depressants.
- Safety net – review again if symptoms not improving after 4–6 weeks.
- For those whose symptoms don't improve after 12 months, consider referring for psychological therapies.

Role play

Information for doctor	Additional information for role player
Patient: Mrs JJ *Age*: 37 years *SH*: Married, 2 children, housewife *PMH*: Asthma *DH*: Salbutamol *Information*: Last consultation 6 months ago due to diarrhoea. No infective cause found. You are a locum GP.	*PC*: "*I've been having problems with my bowels*". *HPC*: Intermittent diarrhoea/constipation for the past month. Some bloating. **No rectal bleeding.** Intermittent lower abdominal pain. No weight loss or mucus in stools. *FH*: Nil. *ICE*: Would like referral to the specialist. *O/E*: Normal abdominal examination.

Gallstones

- Small stones, usually made of cholesterol, which form in the gallbladder.
- Approximately 1 in 3 women and 1 in 6 men will have gallstones at some stage in their lifetime.
- *Figure 5* shows a simple diagram of the gallbladder that can be used to help explain gallstones to your patient.

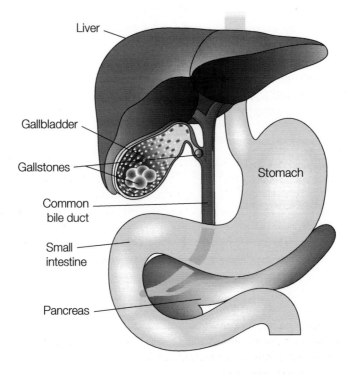

Data gathering

Open question
- *"Can you tell me more about the abdominal pain you've been experiencing?"*

Focused/closed questions

HPC: *"Where exactly is the pain?" "Does it spread anywhere else?" "When did it first start?"*

"What type of pain is it?" "Is the pain intermittent or constant?"

"Does anything make the pain better or worse?"

"Have you had any vomiting or nausea?"

"Have you had any fever?" (red flag)

"Any weight loss or vomiting of blood?" (red flags)

PMH: Any significant medical history?

DH: Are you taking any regular medications? Have you tried any medications to help with the abdominal pain?

FH: Any family history of gallstones or gastrointestinal problems?

SH: Smoking/alcohol/illicit drug history? Occupation?

ICE: *"Do you have any idea what might be causing this abdominal pain?"*

"How does this pain affect you from day to day?"

Examination:
- Temperature, pulse and BP.
- Abdominal examination.

Clinical management

Investigations
- Blood tests – FBC, U&Es, LFTs, CRP, ESR.
- Abdominal ultrasound scan.

Explanation to patient
- Gallstones are formed when some of the chemicals stored in the gallbladder harden to form a mass. It can form one big stone or lots of tiny stones.
- In most cases, gallstones do not cause any symptoms.
- In a small number of cases, gallstones can lead to symptoms due to the stones either becoming trapped in a duct, causing inflammation of the gallbladder, or by moving out into other parts of the body resulting in pain, jaundice (yellow discoloration of the skin) or inflammation of the pancreas.

Management
- Leave alone if causes few or no symptoms.
- Ursodeoxycholic acid – can sometimes dissolve small stones.
- Safety net – review again within 2–3 weeks if symptoms not improving, or sooner if symptoms worsening or the patient develops fever.
- Surgery – cholecystectomy.

Role play

Information for doctor	Additional information for role player
Patient: Mrs CP *Age*: 44 years *SH*: Married, smokes 15 cigs/day, 20 units alcohol/wk. Accountant. *PMH*: Dyspepsia *DH*: Omeprazole 40 mg daily *Information*: Was seen last night by OOH service due to RUQ pain. Was given pain relief and advised to see GP today.	*PC*: Abdominal pain. *HPC*: Intermittent sharp RUQ pain for past few days, which has increased in severity since last night. One episode of vomiting. No fever. Co-codamol helps with the pain. *ICE*: **Worried about what is causing the pain. Would like a scan done.** *O/E*: Abdomen soft, RUQ tenderness. No guarding. No organomegaly or palpable masses.

Chronic kidney disease

- CKD is a common problem which often goes unrecognised, resulting in late referrals to nephrology services (*NICE*, 2008, *CG73: Chronic kidney disease*).
- Those at higher risk of developing CKD should be offered routine testing, including patients with diabetes, hypertension, cardiovascular disease, structural renal tract disease or those with a family history of stage 5 CKD (*NICE*, 2008, *CG73: Chronic kidney disease*).
- There are 5 stages of chronic kidney disease, ranging from mild (stage 1) to severe (stage 5).
- The eGFR (glomerular filtration rate) is now widely accepted as the best overall measure of kidney function.

Data gathering

Open question
- *"What problems have you been experiencing with your kidneys?"*

Focused/closed questions
HPC: *"Have you felt more tired than usual?"*
"Have you noticed any blood in your urine?"
"How many times do you get up at night to pass urine?"
"Have you been passing more urine than usual?"
"Have you noticed any swelling of your feet or ankles?"
"Have you had any shortness of breath, nausea or vomiting?"
"Have you noticed that your skin is more itchy than usual?"
"Have you noticed any weight loss?" (red flag)

PMH: Do you have high blood pressure or diabetes? Have you had any previous problems with your kidneys or heart?

DH: Do you take any regular medications? NSAIDs/ACE inhibitors?

FH: Any family history of kidney problems?

SH: Smoking/alcohol/illicit drug history? Occupation? Who lives with you at home?

ICE: *"What do you think is causing your symptoms?"*

Examination:
- BP.
- Weight.
- Check for anaemia and uraemia.
- Abdominal examination including palpation of kidneys.

Clinical management

Investigations

- Blood test – FBC, U&Es, eGFR, fasting glucose and lipids, HIV/Hep B serology, autoantibodies.
- Check urine for proteinuria (ACR) and blood.
- Renal ultrasound scan.
- Renal biopsy or CT/MRI in secondary care.

Explanation to patient

- The kidneys are two bean-shaped organs which filter out waste products from the blood before converting them into urine. They also help to maintain blood pressure and produce a substance which stimulates red blood cell production.
- Over time, the kidneys become less efficient and this is made worse by diabetes and high blood pressure.

Management (based on *NICE, 2008, CG73: Chronic kidney disease*)

- General lifestyle advice – achieve a healthy weight, exercise, stop smoking, avoid nephrotoxic drugs.
- Aim to keep BP well controlled (consider using ACE inhibitors or angiotensin receptor blockers).
- Reduce CV disease risk (consider statins and aspirin).
- Refer immediately to a specialist if stage 4 or 5 CKD or if any red flags (rapidly declining eGFR, hyperkalaemia, malignant hypertension or suspected renal artery stenosis).
- Also refer to a specialist if stage 3 CKD with a progressive fall in eGFR of >5 ml/year or persistent proteinurea.
- Safety net – return if symptoms worsen.

Stage of CKD	eGFR (ml/min/1.73m²)	Frequency of monitoring
1 (mild)	≥ 90	12 monthly
2	60–89	12 monthly
3a	45–59	6 monthly
3b	30–44	6 monthly
4	15–29	3 monthly
5 (severe)	<15	6 weekly

Role play

Information for doctor	Additional information for role player
Patient: Mrs AB *Age*: 72 years *SH*: Lives with husband, retired. *PMH*: Type 2 diabetes *DH*: Insulin *Information*: Had recent routine blood tests: • urea 18 mmol/l (NR: 4–6) • creatinine 260 mmol/l (NR: 64–111) • eGFR 28 ml/min/1.73 m² Last blood tests 6 months ago: • urea 12 mmol/l • creatinine 170 mmol/l. You are a GP Registrar.	*PC*: *"I was asked to come to discuss my blood test results".* *HPC*: Feels more tired than usual. No haematuria. No ankle oedema. No weight loss. Gets up 2 times at night to pass urine. *ICE*: Worried about her kidneys getting worse. *O/E*: BP 170/95. Slight pallor. Abdominal examination – NAD.

ENT

Hearing loss

- Can be classified as conductive, sensorineural or mixed hearing loss, and may be unilateral or bilateral.
- Can range from mild hearing impairment (27–40 decibels) to profound hearing impairment (>91 decibels)
- Rinne's and Weber's tests can be used to distinguish between conductive and sensorineural hearing loss.

Data gathering

Open question
- *"Can you tell me more about the hearing problems you have been experiencing?"*

Focused/closed questions

HPC: *"When did the hearing problem first start?" "Did it occur suddenly?"*
"Does it affect both ears?"
"What sounds are you able to hear, if any?"
"Have you noticed any ringing in your ears?" (red flag if unilateral)
"Any problem with your balance?" (red flag)
"Have you experienced any pain in your ears?"
"Do you suffer with any dizziness or vertigo?"
"Have you had any previous trauma or injury to your ears?"

PMH: Any previous problems with your ears, or any previous ear operations? Have you had many ear infections in the past? Any history of mumps or meningitis?

DH: Are you taking any regular medications? Have you taken gentamicin in the past?

FH: Is there a family history of hearing problems?

SH: Smoking/alcohol/illicit drug history? Occupation? Who lives with you at home?

ICE: *"Do you have any idea what might be causing the hearing loss?"*
"How has this hearing loss affected life at home and at work?"

Examination:
- Otoscopy.
- Whispered speech test.
- Rinne's and Weber's tests.

Clinical management

Investigations
- Formal hearing test.
- MRI of brain – if indicated.

Explanation to patient
- Conductive deafness results from failure in any of the mechanisms that normally conduct sound waves through the outer ear, the eardrum or the bones of the middle ear.
- Sensorineural deafness results from a problem in the inner ear, especially the cochlea where sound vibrations are converted into nerve signals, or in any part of the brain that subsequently processes these signals.

Management
- Self help – ensure good lighting and sit close to the person you are talking to.
- Wax removal.
- Antibiotics if ear infection.
- Hearing aid or cochlear implants.
- Surgery – for some cases of perforated ear drum or for acoustic neuroma.
- Hearing dogs and assistive devices.
- Safety net – if problem worsening return to GP.
- Further details through Royal National Institute for Deaf People (www.rnid.org.uk)

Role play

Information for doctor	Additional information for role player
Patient: Mrs ED *Age*: 52 years *PMH*: Hysterectomy in 2005 *DH*: Nil *FH*: Nil *Information*: Last consultation was 4 months ago with GP Registrar – right acute otitis media. You are a salaried GP.	*PC*: Decreased hearing in right ear for past couple of months. *HPC*: **No pain in the ear. No tinnitus.** Gradual deterioration. No dizziness or balance problems. **No trauma.** *SH*: School teacher. No FH of hearing problems. *ICE*: Worried about going completely deaf. *O/E*: Decreased hearing on right side. Negative Rinne's test in right ear.

Tinnitus

- Symptom of abnormal noises, usually ringing or buzzing, heard inside the ear.
- The noise does not come from an external source.
- The cause is often not known, but can be a symptom of Ménière's disease or following a head injury or exposure to loud noise.

- Persistent unilateral tinnitus can be caused by an acoustic neuroma.
- There is no cure but there are various ways to reduce the symptoms.

Data gathering

Open question
- *"Can you describe the noises in your ears that you've been experiencing?"*

Focused/closed questions
HPC: *"When did the problem first start?"*
"What specific noises do you hear inside your ear?"
"Do you hear the noises all the time?"
"Do you hear the noises in both ears, or just one?" (red flag if unilateral)
"Are the noises coming from inside the ear or outside?"
"Have you experienced any other symptoms, for example visual changes, dizziness, or problems with balance?" (red flag)
"Any history of injury to the ear?"
"Have you tried anything so far to get rid of the tinnitus?"
PMH: Do you have any medical conditions? Any previous surgery?
DH: Are you on any regular medications?
SH: Smoking/alcohol/illicit drug history? Occupation? Who lives with you at home?
ICE: *"What were you hoping we could do to help?"*
"How has this been affecting you in terms of day to day life?" "Has it stopped you from doing anything you would usually be doing?"
Examination: • Otoscopy.
- Whispered speech test.
- Cranial nerve examination.

Clinical management

Investigations
- Formal hearing test (if indicated).
- Brain MRI scan (if indicated).

Explanation to patient
- The ringing/buzzing noise inside your ear is called tinnitus.
- It is a fairly common problem and is usually temporary.
- It is thought that signals are sent from the ear down the ear nerve to the hearing part of the brain where they are interpreted as noise.
- People often find that the noise is worse at night when you are in a quiet place.

Management

- If caused by a medication then stop this medication.
- SSRIs are sometimes used if associated anxiety and/or depression.
- 'Sound therapy' – having radio or TV on as background noise.
- Hearing aid – if hearing problem.
- Refer to tinnitus clinic.
- Refer to ENT urgently if any suspicion of acoustic neuroma.

Role play

Information for doctor	Additional information for role player
Patient: Mrs LW *Age*: 57 years *SH*: Lives with husband. Housewife. *FH*: Nil *PMH*: Dyspepsia *DH*: Omeprazole 40 mg daily. *Information*: No recent consultations. You are a salaried GP.	*PC*: *"I hear a ringing noise in my ears".* *HPC*: First started about 4 weeks ago. Ringing in both ears. **Noise from inside head. Worse at night. No earache. No visual symptoms. No vomiting or dizziness. No trauma.** Exposure to loud noise at a concert prior to the ringing starting. *ICE*: Would like to know what is causing it and how to get rid of it. *O/E*: Hearing and otoscopy – NAD. Cranial nerves – NAD.

Obstructive sleep apnoea

- Periods of apnoea occur during sleep, when a patient stops breathing for 10 seconds or more.
- As a result of this disturbed sleep, patients often feel tired during the day.
- Most commonly occurs in middle aged, overweight males.
- Smoking, drinking alcohol in the evening, taking sedative drugs and enlarged tonsils are other risk factors.

Data gathering

Open question

- *"Could you tell me a bit more about the breathing problems you've been having at night?"*

Focused/closed questions

HPC: *"When did you first start experiencing these episodes?"*
"How many episodes do you have in a typical night?"
"Has anyone witnessed these episodes?" "What exactly happens?"
"Do you feel tired during the day as a result?"
"Do you usually snore?"
"Do you have difficulty concentrating during the day?"

PMH: Any previous medical problems or any previous ENT surgery?

DH: Do you take any regular medications? Any sleeping tablets?

SH: Smoking/alcohol/illicit drug history? Occupation? Who lives with you at home? Do you drive?

ICE: *"What specific concerns do you have about this sleep problem?"*

Examination: • Weight.

• ENT examination – inspect tonsils and nasal passages.

Clinical management

Investigations

- Epworth sleepiness scale.
- Refer for formal sleep study.

Explanation to patient

- Obstructive sleep apnoea syndrome is a condition where your breathing stops for short spells when you are asleep.
- It occurs because the throat muscles relax and become so floppy that they cause a temporary blockage of the airway. It usually wakes you up due to the decreased blood oxygen level and then when you start breathing again you will normally go off to sleep again.

Management

- General measures – weight loss if overweight, decrease alcohol intake and stop smoking, and sleep on side.
- Mandibular advancement device for mild OSAS.
- Safety net – return if above measures not helping.
- CPAP for moderate to severe OSAS.
- Surgery – adeno-tonsillectomy if large tonsils or adenoids.
- DVLA – must inform DVLA and must not drive if you have OSAS.

Role play

Information for doctor	Additional information for role player
Patient: Mr JH	*PC*: *"My wife is concerned about my snoring".*
Age: 62 years	*HPC*: *"She also said that I stop breathing in the night periodically".* 2–3 episodes per night. **Tiredness during the day.**
SH: Unemployed, lives with wife	
PMH: COPD, obesity	*SH*: Smokes 20 cigs/day. Alcohol 40 units/week.
DH: Seretide, symbicort	*ICE*: **Would like something to stop the snoring.**
Information: Last seen 1 month ago for COPD review. You are a salaried GP.	*O/E*: Weight 110 kg (BMI 37), throat – NAD.

Ophthalmology

Red eye

- Red eye is a relatively common presentation in primary care, most of which are due to quite trivial causes.
- Causes of painful red eye include acute angle closure glaucoma, keratitis, trauma and acute anterior uveitis.
- Causes of painless red eye include conjunctivitis, episcleritis and subconjunctival haemorrhage.

Data gathering

Open question
- "Can you tell me more about your eye symptoms?"

Focused/closed questions

HPC: *"When did the problem first start?"*
"Have your symptoms got worse since then?"
"Is the eye painful? If so, how severe?" (red flag if severe pain)
"Is your vision affected?"
"Did you get a sudden loss of vision?" (red flag)
"Any watering or itchiness of the eye?"
"Any trauma or contact with chemicals in the eye?" (red flag)
"Have you noticed that your eye is more sensitive to the light?"
"Have you suffered from any headache, vomiting, rash, fever?" (red flags)
"Any contact with other people with red/sticky eyes?"
"Do you wear contact lenses?"

PMH: Do you have any medical conditions, e.g. diabetes?
Any previous eye problems or eye surgery?

SH: Smoking/alcohol/illicit drug history? Occupation? Exposure to chemicals?

FH: Any FH of eye problems?

ICE: *"Do you have any idea what might be causing these eye problems?"*

Examination:
- Inspection of the eye including sclera and lids (can use fluoroscein drops).
- Visual acuity, visual fields and eye movements.
- Pupil reflexes.
- Systems examination if suspecting systemic cause.

Clinical management

Investigations
- Slit lamp examination.

Explanation to patient
- There are numerous different causes of red eye, which can be categorised into painful and painless.
- Some cases require urgent treatment, and it is therefore important to be able to distinguish between the different causes.

Management
- Same day ophthalmology referral if moderate to severe eye pain, reduced visual acuity, unilateral red eye, abnormal pupillary reactions or suspected penetrating trauma injury.
- Safety net – in all other cases if no improvement in symptoms over the next few days return to the GP.

Acute painful red eye
- Acute angle closure glaucoma (severe pain, haloes around lights, vomiting). Signs include decreased visual acuity, hazy cornea, fixed semi-dilated pupil. Refer immediately.
- Acute anterior uveitis (photophobia, blurred vision, headache). Signs include decreased visual acuity, red eye, constricted or irregular pupil. Refer within 24 hours.
- Trauma to eye – painful eye. Refer immediately if risk of serious trauma.

Acute non-painful red eye
- Conjunctivitis (mild discomfort, discharge from eye). Signs include normal visual acuity and unilateral or bilateral discharge. Treat with chloramphenicol or sodium cromoglycate.
- Subconjunctival haemorrhage (spontaneous or traumatic). Signs include normal visual acuity with blood under conjunctiva. Usually self resolving. Check BP.

Role play

Information for doctor	Additional information for role player
Patient: Mr GR	*PC*: "*I've got a pain in my right eye*".
Age: 36 years	*HPC*: Pain started this morning. Also red eye. No trauma. No fever. Vision decreased in right eye. No headache or vomiting.
SH: Lives with wife and 3 children. Builder.	
PMH: Crohn's disease	
DH: Sulfasalazine	*ICE*: Worried about going blind.
Information: Called the surgery this morning requesting an urgent appointment due to eye symptoms. You are a GP Partner.	*O/E*: Injection around the right iris and photophobia in the right eye when a direct light is shone.

Neurology

Headache

- The SIGN 2008 guidelines define headaches as follows:
  - Primary headache disorders: not associated with underlying pathology, e.g. tension headache, cluster headaches, migraines.
  - Secondary headache disorders: headache attributed to underlying pathology, e.g. from infection, neoplasm or drug induced.
  - Chronic headache: >15 days per month for more than 3 months.
- The commonest type of headache seen in primary care is a tension-type headache.

Data gathering

Open question
- *"Can you tell me more about your headache?"*

Focused/closed questions

HPC: *"Where exactly are you experiencing the pain?" "Does the pain spread anywhere else?"*
"When did it first start? Is it a constant or intermittent pain?"
"How severe is the pain?"
"Any nausea, vomiting, visual symptoms or rash?" (red flags)
"Is it worse at any particular time of the day?"
"Was the headache of sudden onset?" (red flag)
"Have you had any seizures or noticed any personality changes?" (red flags)

PMH: Any past history of migraines/headaches?

FH: Any family history of migraine?

SH: Smoking/alcohol/illicit drug history? Occupation? Stress? Who lives with you at home?

ICE: *"What worries you about this headache?"*
"How is this headache affecting your daily activities?"

Examination:
- BP.
- Neurological examination including cranial nerves.
- Fundoscopy.

Clinical management

Investigations
- Not routinely required.
- Brain MRI if suspected brain pathology.

Explanation to patient
- Tension headaches – typically the pain is around the 'hat-band' area. Can be described as a squeezing or pressure on the head. Usually on both sides of the head, and usually lasts a few hours. Often caused by stress or physical tension.
- Cluster headaches – pain typically lasts 45–90 minutes and attacks usually occur one to two times daily. The clusters of headaches usually last from a few weeks to a few months. The pain is centred around or behind the eye, temple or forehead and is unilateral. The pain is often accompanied by watering of the eye on the same side, runny nose or nasal congestion.

Management (based on *SIGN*, 2008, *107: Diagnosis and management of headaches in adults*)
- Headache diary.
- Tension headache: try to eliminate stressors, exercise, paracetamol, NSAIDs, amitriptylline.
- Cluster headache: oxygen and sumatriptan for an acute attack. Prophylaxis includes melatonin and verapamil (both unlicensed).
- Safety net – if not improving to return to GP.
- If suspected brain pathology refer to neurology urgently (focal neurology, reduced GCS).

Role play

Information for doctor	Additional information for role player
Patient: Mr BA *Age*: 28 years *SH*: Investment banker *FH*: Nil *PMH*: Nil *DH*: Nil *Information*: Recent consultation with locum GP due to headaches. Neurological examination – NAD. You are a GP Partner.	*PC*: "*I saw one of the other doctors recently due to headaches but they're not getting any better*". *HPC*: Headaches occurring every day. Pain mainly across forehead. No visual symptoms. No nausea or vomiting. Has been very busy at work and under quite a lot of stress. Recently broke up with girlfriend. *ICE*: Would like some painkillers for the headache as paracetamol and Nurofen not helping. *O/E*: BP 110/70 mmHg. Fundoscopy – NAD.

Migraine

- A condition causing severe headache often with associated nausea, vomiting or visual symptoms.
- Between migraine attacks the symptoms completely resolve.
- The two main types of migraine are classic migraine (migraine with aura) and common migraine (migraine without aura).

Data gathering

Open question
- *"Can you tell me more about your headache?"*

Focused/closed questions

HPC: *"Where exactly is the location of the pain?"*
"Do you get any associated nausea or vomiting with the headache?"
"Is the headache worse at any particular time of the day?"
"Do you get any visual symptoms or pins and needles associated with the headache?"
"Is there any warning prior to the onset of the headache?"
"Are there any particular triggers or any aggravating factors?"
"Any relieving factors?"
"Have you noticed any problems with your balance or co-ordination?" (possible red flag)

PMH: Have you suffered from migraines in the past?

DH: Are you on any regular medications? Do you take the combined contraceptive pill?

FH: Any FH of headaches/migraines?

SH: Smoking/alcohol/illicit drug history? Occupation? Stress?

ICE: *"Do you have any thoughts as to what is causing these headaches?"*

Examination:
- BP.
- Neurological examination including cranial nerves.
- Fundoscopy.

Clinical management

Investigations
- No specific investigations (clinical diagnosis).
- Only if ruling out other causes of headaches, e.g. CT brain to rule out intracranial bleed or tumour.

Explanation to patient
- The pain of a migraine is thought to occur when excited nerve cells trigger a nerve in the head to release chemicals that irritate and cause swelling of the blood vessels

on the surface of the brain. These swollen vessels then send pain signals to an area of the brain that processes pain information.

- There are two types of migraine – a classical migraine which is when you have a warning sign, known as an aura, before the migraine begins, and a common migraine when there is no warning sign.

Management

- Simple analgesia/NSAIDs.
- Anti-emetics.
- Triptans – they cause the blood vessels around the brain to constrict. This reverses the widening of blood vessels which is believed to be part of the migraine process.
- Prevention – avoid triggers. Beta-blockers or amitriptyline can also be used.
- Safety net – refer if uncertain diagnosis or not controlled with above treatments.

Role play

Information for doctor	Additional information for role player
Patient: Ms JB *Age*: 25 years *SH*: Lives with friends. Postgraduate student *FH*: Nil *PMH*: Nil *DH*: Microgynon *Information*: You are a GP Registrar.	*PC*: "*I've recently been getting very bad headaches*". *HPC*: Three episodes of bad headaches in the past month. Last for approx 1 day. Pain on left side of head. **Also had some numbness of the face prior to the headache. No visual symptoms.** No vomiting but nausea. Paracetamol not helping. *ICE*: **Worried it may be related to the contraceptive pill.** *O/E*: Neurological exam – NAD, fundoscopy – NAD.

Multiple sclerosis

- MS is a disorder of the central nervous system resulting in damage to the nerve fibres that carry messages to and from the brain.
- Symptoms can occur in any part of the body, and include numbness, tingling, blurring of vision, muscle weakness and problems with mobility/balance.
- Symptoms can initially come and go, and then usually with time become permanent.
- Thought to be an auto-immune cause, resulting in inflammation of the myelin sheath around the nerve fibre.
- There are three main types – relapsing remitting, primary progressive or secondary progressive.

Data gathering

Open question

- *"Can you tell me what symptoms have you been experiencing?"*

Focused/closed questions

HPC: *"When did these symptoms first start?"*
"Have you experienced any weakness/numbness/balance problems/ visual symptoms?"
"Have you had any problems with your speech?"
"Have you had any problems with controlling your bowels or bladder?"
"Have you had any problems with muscle spasms or mobility?"
"Are these symptoms constant or intermittent?" "Are they worsening?"

PMH: Any history of any medical conditions?

FH: Any family history of neurological problems or MS?

DH: Do you take any regular medications?

SH: Who lives with you at home? Smoking/alcohol/illicit drug history? Occupation?

ICE: *"How are you managing at home with these symptoms?"*

Examination:
- Neurological examination including cranial nerves
- Eye examination

Clinical management

Investigations

- MRI of brain.
- Visual evoked potential studies.
- Lumbar puncture.

Explanation to patient

- Patches of inflammation occur in parts of the brain or spinal cord, and the nerve fibres stop working properly, resulting in symptoms.

Management (based on *NICE, 2003, CG8: Multiple sclerosis*)

- If suspected MS refer to neurology for confirmatory diagnosis.
- No cure.
- For acute episodes of MS with disabling symptoms – high dose methylprednisolone for 3–5 days.
- Immunomodulatory agents, e.g. beta-interferon – can reduce the number of relapses.
- Other medications, e.g. anti-spasmodics, anti-depressants and anti-cholinergics.
- Physiotherapy, occupational therapy, speech therapy, psychological therapy.
- Safety net – return to GP if symptoms not improving within 1–2 weeks.

Role play

Information for doctor	Additional information for role player
Patient: Ms SC *Age*: 37 years *SH*: Lives alone. Receptionist. *PMH*: Polycystic ovarian syndrome *DH*: Nil *Information*: No recent consultations. You are a salaried GP.	*PC*: *"I seem to be more unsteady on my feet, and fell over yesterday".* *HPC*: 4-week history of problems with balance. Not improving. **Also blurring of vision in left eye and pain behind left eye.** No earache. No headache. No numbness but muscle weakness in both legs. **No bowel or bladder symptoms. No speech problems.** *FH*: Nil *ICE*: Worried about a brain tumour. *O/E*: Fundoscopy – blurring of left optic disc. Neurological examination – decreased sensation in left leg. Power decreased in lower limbs bilaterally.

Temporal arteritis

- Condition of unknown aetiology, causing inflammation of the large and medium arteries of the head, most commonly the temporal artery.
- It is an uncommon condition, mainly affecting people over the age of 60.
- Can lead to serious conditions such as blindness and stroke.
- Symptoms include headache, jaw pain, scalp tenderness and visual disturbances.
- Up to half of people with temporal arteritis will develop a related condition called polymyalgia rheumatica (PMR).

Data gathering

Open question
- *"Can you tell me more about the symptoms you've been experiencing?"*

Focused/closed questions
HPC: *"When did these symptoms first start?"*
"Have your symptoms worsened since then?"
"Was it a sudden onset?"
"Have you experienced any headache, jaw pain, numbness or visual disturbances?"
"Do you have any tiredness or muscle weakness?"
PMH: Do you have any medical conditions?
DH: Do you take any regular medications?
SH: Who lives with you at home? Smoking/alcohol history?

ICE: *"What were you hoping we could do to help?"*

Examination: • Palpation of head – prominence of temporal artery, tenderness +/- pulsation.
              • Fundoscopy – possible ischaemia.

Clinical management

Investigations
• Blood test – ESR, CRP, platelets.
• Temporal artery biopsy.

Explanation to patient
• Condition caused by inflammation of the arteries on the side of the head.

Management
• Refer to secondary care if temporal arteritis is suspected.
• High dose steroids (40–60 mg prednisolone, tapering down over several months).
• Low dose aspirin.
• Safety net – if symptoms not improving return to GP.

Role play

Information for doctor	Additional information for role player
Patient: Mr GA *Age*: 63 years *SH*: Lives with wife. Retired. *FH*: Nil *DH*: Nil *PMH*: Bowel cancer in 2007. Had subtotal colectomy. *Information*: You are a GP Registrar	*PC*: *"I've been experiencing sharp pains around my eyes".* *HPC*: Started this morning. Normal visual acuity. Shooting pains around temples. **Very sensitive to touch. No muscle weakness or lethargy.** Intermittent jaw pain, mainly while eating. *ICE*: Very worried at what is causing it. *O/E*: Temporal artery tenderness. Normal visual acuity. Fundoscopy normal.

Transient ischaemic attack

• Temporary lack of blood supply to the brain, resulting in symptoms similar to a stroke, but which resolve within 24 hours.
• Most commonly caused by a small blood clot, and is sometimes referred to as a 'mini stroke'.
• Treatment includes reducing any risk factors for developing a stroke, and medication to reduce the risk of blood clotting.

Data gathering

Open question

- *"Can you tell me more about the symptoms you have been experiencing?"*

Focused/closed questions

HPC: *"Have you experienced any weakness of your face, arms or legs? If so, which side is affected?"*
"Do you have any problems with your speech, swallowing or vision?"
"Any numbness or pins and needles in any part of your body?"
"Have the symptoms improved since they first started?"
"Have you had any dizziness or loss of balance?"
"Have you had any loss of consciousness, confusion or seizures?"
(red flags)

PMH: Any previous history of TIA, stroke or heart problems? Any previous heart operations? Do you have high blood pressure or diabetes?

DH: Do you take any regular medications?

FH: Do you have any family history of diabetes, heart disease or stroke?

SH: Who lives with you at home? Support? Smoking/alcohol/illicit drug history? Occupation?

ICE: *"Do you have any ideas as to what is causing your symptoms?"*

Examination:
- BP and pulse (rate and rhythm).
- Cardiovascular system – check for heart murmurs and carotid bruits.
- Neurological examination and cranial nerves: check for weakness, visual loss and gait.

Clinical management

Investigations

- ECG – to check for atrial fibrillation.
- Blood test – FBC, fasting glucose, cholesterol (to check for risk factors).
- Coagulation studies – may be required, but should be discussed with a specialist first.
- Echocardiogram – if suspecting cardiac valve problem.
- Doppler ultrasound scan of carotids, or MRI/CT brain – only if requested by a specialist.

Explanation to patient

- A TIA produces a group of symptoms which occur due to a temporary lack of blood to part of the brain. This usually happens due to a tiny blood clot blocking a small blood vessel in the brain, stopping the blood flow and starving part of the brain of oxygen. It usually only blocks the blood flow for a few minutes and then recovers back to normal. It is considered as a 'warning sign' that you are at higher risk of having a stroke or heart attack.
- You are at higher risk of a TIA or a stroke if you are overweight, smoke, have high blood pressure, high cholesterol or diabetes.

Management (*NICE, 2008, CG68: Stroke*)

- In people with sudden onset of neurological symptoms, a validated tool such as FAST (face, arm, speech test) should be used to screen for the diagnosis of a stroke or TIA.
- People with a suspected TIA who are at high risk of a stroke (e.g. an ABCD^2 score* of 4 or above) should receive immediate aspirin 300 mg daily, specialist assessment within 24 hours of the onset of symptoms, and commencement of secondary prevention as soon as the diagnosis is confirmed.
- People with an ABCD2 score of 3 or below should have aspirin 300 mg daily (NICE do not state how long the aspirin at 300 mg dose should be continued after a TIA) started immediately and a specialist assessment as soon as possible but definitely within 1 week.
- Reduce any risk factors, e.g. stop smoking, control high blood pressure, treat high cholesterol and atrial fibrillation, weight loss and exercise.
- Patients with more than one TIA in a week should be investigated in hospital immediately.
- Inform DVLA – patient must not drive for 1 month.
- Safety net – routinely review in the GP surgery within 1 week even if all the TIA symptoms have now resolved.

*ABCD^2 – scoring system to assess for high risk TIAs, taking into account **a**ge, **b**lood pressure, **c**linical features, **d**uration of symptoms and whether the patient is **d**iabetic (see *NICE, 2008, CG68: Stroke*).

Role play

Information for doctor	Additional information for role player
Patient: Mrs FY *Age*: 74 years old *SH*: Retired, lives with husband *PMH*: NIDDM *DH*: Metformin 850 mg TDS *Information*: Last consultation 2 weeks ago with practice nurse – BP 180/98 mmHg, BMI 34. You are a GP Registrar.	*PC*: Woke up this morning with slurred speech and weakness of left arm which has now resolved. **No visual symptoms. No headache or dizziness.** No LOC or seizures. *ICE*: Concerned about a stroke as her husband had a stroke a few years ago. *O/E*: Neuro exam – NAD. Heart rate regular. BP 170/95 mmHg.

Rheumatology/ musculoskeletal

Back pain

- About 80% of people will have at least one bout of back pain in their lifetime.
- 'Non-specific' back pain is the most common type.
- Other causes of back pain include sciatica, cauda equina syndrome, ankylosing spondylitis and arthritis.

Data gathering

Open question
- *"Can you tell me more about the back pain you have been experiencing?"*

Focused/closed questions

HPC: *"When did the pain first start?" "Was there any injury or trauma?"*
"Where is the pain?" "Does the pain radiate anywhere else?"
"Is the pain constant?"
"Is the pain worse at any particular time of the day or night?"
"What type of pain is it?"
"Are you able to walk?"
"Have you been experiencing any numbness or tingling of the legs or around the back passage?" (red flag)
"Have you ever lost control of your bowels or bladder?" (red flag)
"Any fever or weight loss?" (red flag)

PMH: Any history of back problems?

FH: Any family history of back problems?

DH: Are you taking any medications at present?

SH: Occupation? Who lives with you at home?

ICE: *"How has this pain been affecting you at home and at work?"*

Examination:
- Back examination including straight leg raise (see *Appendix 1*).
- Sensation and reflexes.

Clinical management

Investigations
- No investigations required for non-specific back pain.
- Consider lumbo-sacral spinal X-ray/MRI if considering other causes.

Explanation to patient
- Non-specific low back pain means that the pain is not due to any specific cause or underlying disease that can be found.
- In some cases the cause may be a sprain of a ligament or muscle, or a minor problem with a disc between two vertebrae (back bones).
- These causes of back pain are impossible to prove by tests, however.

Management
- Exercise.
- Analgesia – paracetamol +/- NSAIDs, increasing to codeine or tramadol if required.
- Muscle relaxant – consider diazepam for short term use.
- Physiotherapy.
- Social – sick note, driving.
- Refer immediately if any signs of cauda equina syndrome.
- Refer to orthopaedics or pain clinic if persistent non-specific back pain not responding to the above treatments.
- Safety net – return if not improving.

NICE recommendations (2009, CG88: Low back pain)
Recommendations for chronic non-specific back pain include:
- Tricyclic anti-depressants, e.g. amitriptyline.
- Structured exercise programme.
- Manual therapy – several sessions of massage, spinal mobilisation and/or spinal manipulation.
- Also consider acupuncture, CBT and/or referral to a pain clinic.

Role play

Information for doctor	Additional information for role player
Patient: Mr AK *Age*: 58 years *SH*: Lives with wife, works as builder *PMH*: Epilepsy *DH*: Phenytoin *Information*: You are a GP Partner.	*PC*: "I've got really bad lower back pain". *HPC*: Back pain for 1 week. Slipped on concrete at work. **No radiation of pain down legs. No numbness/tingling in legs. No urinary/bowel symptoms.** Pain constant but worse when moving. *ICE*: Would like an X-ray of his back and painkillers. *O/E*: Tenderness on flexion of back. Straight leg raise >50°, reflexes and sensation normal.

Shoulder pain

- The most common causes of shoulder pain seen in primary care are frozen shoulder, rotator cuff disorders, osteoarthritis and shoulder instability.
- Frozen shoulder (adhesive capsulitis) occurs when there is thickening, swelling and tightening of the tissues surrounding the shoulder joint. This results in decreased movement of the shoulder.
- The rotator cuff is a group of muscles around the shoulder joint which provides stability and movement of the shoulder. The rotator cuff can be affected by a tear, tendonitis or bursitis.
- Shoulder pain can also be caused by extrinsic causes, for example, polymyalgia rheumatica or referred pain from other structures such as the neck, heart or gallbladder.

Data gathering

Open question
- *"Can you tell me more about your shoulder pain?"*

Focused/closed questions

HPC: *"When did the pain first start?"*
"Which shoulder is affected?" "Are you left/right handed?"
"Did you injure your shoulder?"
"Where exactly is the pain?" "Does the pain spread anywhere?"
"Do you have decreased movement in the shoulder?"
"Do you get any pain at night?" (red flag)
"Do you have pain at rest or only on movement?"
"Does the pain restrict activities?"
"Have you noticed any weight loss, lumps or swelling?" "Any fever or redness over the shoulder?" "Any numbness?" (red flags)

PMH: Any previous shoulder problems, or past surgery?
Any history of diabetes, cancer or ischaemic heart disease?

DH: Do you take any regular medications?

SH: Who lives with you at home? How are you coping at home? Occupation? Do you drive? Do you play any regular sports?

ICE: *"What were you expecting in terms of treatment for your shoulder problem?"*

Examination: • Shoulder examination (see *Appendix 1*).

Clinical management

Investigations
- Shoulder X-ray – if suspected bony injury.
- Shoulder MRI – if suspecting rotator cuff/soft tissue problem.

- Shoulder arthroscopy.
- Blood test – FBC, ESR, CRP (if red flag symptoms).

Explanation to patient

The commonest causes of shoulder pain are described below:

Common causes of shoulder pain	*Description*	*History*	*Examination*	*Explanation to patient*	*Management*
Rotator cuff tendinopathy	Degenerative changes of the tendons around the shoulder joint. Commonest cause of shoulder pain.	History of repetitive movement or heavy lifting.	Painful arc. Pain on active/ resisted movement; impingement.	Damage to the tissues that connect the muscles to bones at the shoulder joint.	Activity modification. Analgesia/ NSAIDs, steroid injections, physiotherapy, surgery.
Rotator cuff tear	The rotator cuff is a group of four muscles and their tendons, providing shoulder stability. A tear is usually due to trauma. Most common in >40 age group.	Pain and weakness of shoulder.	Shoulder weakness. Unable to raise arm over head.	Tear to one or more of the four tendons of the rotator cuff muscles.	Analgesia, rest, orthopaedic referral for acute tear.
Adhesive capsulitis	Otherwise known as frozen shoulder. Can take up to 3 years to resolve. More common in 40–60 year age group and in diabetics.	Restricted shoulder movement and stiffness. Pain deep in joint.	Tenderness on palpation of shoulder joint. Decreased ROM of shoulder.	The tissues surrounding the shoulder joint become inflamed and stiff, restricting shoulder movement.	Analgesia/ NSAIDs, steroid injection, physiotherapy, surgery.
Osteoarthritis	Inflammation of the shoulder joint.	Gradual onset of pain, stiffness and decreased movement of shoulder joint.	Tenderness on palpation of shoulder joint. Muscle weakness. Crepitus. Decreased ROM.	Due to wear and tear of the shoulder joint.	Analgesia/ NSAIDs, steroid injection, physiotherapy, surgery.

Further management

- Refer urgently if suspected fracture, dislocation, nerve damage or red flags.
- Safety net – return to GP if not improving.
- Routine referral to orthopaedics for consideration of surgery/arthroscopy if non-surgical measures unsuccessful.

Role play

Information for doctor	Additional information for role player
Patient: Mr DF *Age*: 39 years *SH*: Lives alone. Unemployed. Smokes 20 cigs/day. Drinks 40 units alcohol/week. *FH*: Nil *PMH*: Nil *Information*: You are a salaried GP.	*PC*: *"I've done something to my shoulder".* *HPC*: Fell on left shoulder 6 weeks ago. Did improve but now has decreased movement of left shoulder. **Very painful around shoulder joint.** Pain mainly on movement. No swelling or numbness. **No night pain.** *ICE*: Would like to know the cause and would like painkillers. *O/E*: Tender on palpation around shoulder joint. Decreased abduction and internal rotation of shoulder. No swelling.

Knee pain

- Common causes of knee pain include meniscal, ligamentous or joint problems (osteoarthritis/rheumatoid arthritis/gout).
- Other common problems include patellar tendonitis, chondromalacia patellae, baker's cyst and Osgood–Schlatter disease.

Data gathering

Open question

- *"Can you describe in more detail the knee pain you've been experiencing?"*

Focused/closed questions

HPC: *"Where exactly are you experiencing the pain?" "Does the pain spread anywhere else?"*
"When did the pain first start?" " Is it getting worse?"
"Is the pain worse at any particular time of the day?"
"Is there anything which makes the pain better or worse?"
"Did you injure your knee?"
"Does your knee ever lock or give way?"
"Is there any swelling of your knee?"
"Are you still able to walk or run?"
"Do you have a fever?" (red flag)

PMH: Any previous knee problems or surgery?

FH: Any FH of joint problems?

SH: Who lives with you at home? Stairs at home? Occupation?

DH: *"Have you tried any painkillers for the pain so far?"*

ICE: *"Is there anything in particular you were hoping we could do to help?"*
"How does this pain affect you at home or at work?"

Examination: • Knee examination (see *Appendix 1*).

Clinical management

Investigations
- Blood tests – FBC, ESR, CRP, calcium, RhF.
- Fluid from knee aspirate for microscopy.
- Knee X-ray.
- Knee MRI.
- Refer for knee arthroscopy.

Explanation to patient and management

Common causes of knee pain	*Description*	*History*	*Examination*	*Explanation to patient*	*Management*
Osteoarthritis	Inflammation of the joints.	Gradual onset of pain, stiffness and limitation of joint movement.	Possible deformity and swelling of knee, decreased ROM, crepitus, decreased function.	Caused by wear and tear of the knee joint.	See Osteoarthritis section.
Meniscal problem	Damage to the menisci which help to lubricate and stabilise the knee joint.	Knee locking/ giving way. Medial or lateral knee pain. Often due to twisting injury.	Knee swelling +/- effusion. Decreased extension of knee. Pain or 'clicking' on twisting the knee during extension.	Menisci act like shock absorbers in the knee; can be torn commonly by a forceful twisting injury.	Analgesia +/- NSAIDs. Small tears may heal themselves. Larger tears require surgery.
Ligamentous injury	There are four ligaments which provide stability to the knee. These can be stretched, torn or ruptured usually by a forceful injury.	Pain, swelling and instability of the knee. Popping or snapping sound at the time of injury.	Swelling and tenderness around the knee joint. Effusion in knee. Decreased ROM. Anterior/ posterior draw test and Lachman test may be +ve.	Ligaments are strong tissues around joints which connect bone together. Ligaments can be injured usually by being stretched during a sudden pull.	Analgesia/ NSAIDs. Rest, immobilisation, physiotherapy, surgery.
Patellar tendonitis	Inflammation of the patellar tendon where it attaches to the patella. Can progress to tearing and degeneration of the tendon.	Pain over the patella usually due to overuse injury from repetitive overloading, e.g. jumping.	Knee swelling. Patellar tenderness on palpation. Pain on extension/ flexion of the knee.	Inflammation of the fibrous tissue that connects muscle to bone around the knee cap.	Rest, activity modification, NSAIDs, strengthening exercises, steroid joint injection.

Common causes of knee pain	Description	History	Examination	Explanation to patient	Management
Chondro-malacia patellae	Softening of articular cartilage of the patella.	Common in young girls. Usually due to indirect trauma. Usually anterior knee pain worse on rising and using stairs.	Patellar tenderness, crepitus, fluid behind the knee. Pain on passive movements of the knee.	Irritation of the undersurface of the knee cap.	Avoid repetitive knee bending and excessive activity. Immobilisation, analgesia/ NSAIDs, knee supports, surgery.
Osgood–Schlatter's	Inflammation of the tibial tubercle due to overuse and excessive force acting on this bone.	Occurs in teenagers, especially boys. Pain and swelling just below the knee, worse after activity and eases with rest.	Tender bony lump and swelling below the knee cap. Normal ROM.	Bony protrusion below the knee becomes inflamed.	Ease off strenuous sport, ice pack, knee support, simple analgesia, physiotherapy.
Baker's cyst	Benign swelling of the semi-membranous bursa behind the knee joint.	Pain and swelling at the back of the knee. Knee locking.	Transilluminable swelling in the popliteal space.	Fluid-filled swelling that develops at the back of the knee.	May self resolve with no treatment or NSAIDs. RICE. Occasionally steroid injection or surgery.

Role play

Information for doctor	Additional information for role player
Patient: Mrs SK *Age*: 58 years *SH*: Lives with husband. Has stairs at home. *FH*: Diabetes *PMH*: Diabetes *DH*: Metformin, gliclazide *Information*: You are a locum GP.	*PC*: "*I've got terrible pain in my right knee*". *HPC*: Right knee pain for the past few weeks. No trauma. Pain over patella and medial side. **Worse after walking. Knee sometimes gives way. No locking.** *ICE*: Would like a scan and would like some stronger painkillers. *O/E*: No swelling or effusion. Tenderness around medial joint line. Some crepitus on flexion of knee. Normal ROM. Decreased extension of right knee.

Osteoarthritis

- Inflammation of the joints resulting in pain and stiffness.
- Commonly affects hips, knees and hands.
- Treatment includes analgesia, physiotherapy or surgery (joint replacement).

Data gathering

Open question
- *"Can you tell me more about the pain you've been experiencing?"*

Focused/closed questions
HPC: *"Where exactly is the pain?" "Does the pain spread anywhere else?"*
"When did it start?" "Is it getting worse?"
"Is the pain worse at any particular time of the day?"
"Are any other joints affected?"
"Does anything make the pain better/worse?"
"Any fever or weight loss?" (red flags)

PMH: Any previous injuries or joint problems?

FH: Any FH of arthritis?

SH: Smoking/alcohol history? Occupation? Who lives with you at home?

ICE: *"What do you think is causing this pain?"*
"How is it impacting on your quality of life?"

Examination: • Joint examination.

Clinical management

Investigations
- X-ray.

Explanation to patient
- A joint is where two bones meet, and there is a hard smooth tissue called cartilage which covers the ends of the bones at the joint. There is also a fluid surrounding the joint called synovial fluid that helps to lubricate the joint.
- In osteoarthritis, the joint cartilage becomes damaged and worn, and the bone around the cartilage can also be damaged.

Management (based on *NICE*, 2008, *CG59: Osteoarthritis*)
- Conservative management – weight loss, exercise, walking aids, sensible footwear, splints/braces.
- Analgesia +/– NSAIDs, topical capsaicin.
- Heat/cold packs.
- Intra-articular steroid injections.

- Physiotherapy +/- occupational therapy.
- Safety net – return if symptoms not improving.
- Refer for surgery if non-surgical treatments have failed.
- NICE currently does not recommend glucosamine, although some people find this improves their symptoms.

Role play

Information for doctor	Additional information for role player
Patient: Mrs PS	*PC*: *"I have come to discuss my hip X-ray results".*
Age: 73 years	*HPC*: Left hip pain which is mainly worse at the end
SH: Lives in a residential home.	of the day after walking. **No radiation down**
PMH: Blindness, hypertension.	**the leg. Affects ability to walk.** No other joints
DH: Bendrofluazide 2.5 mg OD.	affected. **No weight loss or fever.** No trauma.
Information: Last consultation 2 weeks ago – left hip	*FH*: Nil.
pain for several months. X-ray left hip –	*ICE*: Hoping for some painkillers and wants to know
joint space narrowing, osteophytes.	diagnosis.

Osteoporosis

- Occurs when a person's bones are less dense than normal and more prone to fractures.
- About 1 in 3 women over the age of 50 are thought to have osteoporosis.
- Risk factors include early menopause, family history, low body mass index, smokers, patients on long-term steroids and those who have a sedentary lifestyle.
- Diagnosis is established using a DEXA scan and management includes bisphosphonates and lifestyle measures.

Data gathering

Open questions
- *"What problems have you been experiencing with your bones?"*
- *"What do you understand about your recent DEXA scan results?"*

Focused/closed questions
HPC: *"Have you ever fractured any bones before?"*
"Do you have any bone pains?"
"Have you had any recent falls?"
"At what age did you go through the menopause?"
"Have you noticed any weight loss or night sweats?" (red flags)
PMH: *"Do you have any history of bone problems?"* *"Do you have any illnesses such as diabetes or inflammatory bowel disease?"*
FH: *"Is there a history of osteoporosis or hip fractures in your family?"*

DH: Are you on any regular medications? Have you ever been on long term steroids?

SH: Smoking/alcohol history? Diet/exercise?

ICE: *"What concerns do you have about your bones?"*

Examination:
- BMI.
- Examine bone/joint if pain.

Clinical management

Investigations
- DEXA scan.
- Blood test – FBC, U&Es, TFTs, calcium, phosphate, vitamin D, LFTs, ALP, LH, FSH, testosterone.

Explanation to patient
- A DEXA scan compares a patient's bone density to the population mean density (e.g. young adults of the same sex). The results are expressed as a standard deviation from the mean.
- If your DEXA scan result is between 0 and −1, this implies that you have a normal bone density.
- If your DEXA scan result is between −1 and −2.5, this implies that you have osteopenia (slightly weaker bones than normal).
- If your DEXA scan result is less than −2.5, this implies that you have osteoporosis.

Management
- Conservative management – increase dietary calcium intake and increase weight bearing exercise.
- Stop smoking.
- Consider reducing or stopping steroids if on steroid therapy.
- Calcium and vitamin D.
- Consider HRT (no longer first line).

NICE Recommendations for primary and secondary prevention of osteoporosis *(NICE, 2008, TA160/161: Osteoporosis)*
- Alendronate is recommended as first line if the patient fulfils the criteria for treatment (confirmed osteoporosis with a risk factor for fracture or if fragility fracture over 75 years).
- Risedronate and etidronate can be used when alendronate cannot be tolerated, and if these cannot be tolerated then strontium ranelate can be used (or also raloxifene for secondary prevention).

Role play

Information for doctor	Additional information for role player
Patient: Mrs ER *Age*: 64 years *PMH*: Breast cancer *DH*: Nil *Information*: Had a DEXA scan 2 weeks ago. Results – spinal T score 1.1; hip T score – 2.8.	*PC*: "*I have come for the results of my bone scan I had recently*". *HPC*: Had a Colles fracture 2 months ago following a fall. No bone pain at present. Reached menopause aged 54 years. *FH*: **Mum and sister had osteoporosis.** *ICE*: Thinks she may have osteoporosis so keen to start taking medication to protect the bones as this is what her sister took.

Rheumatoid arthritis

- Common form of arthritis resulting in pain, swelling and inflammation of the joints.
- Most commonly develops between the ages of 40 and 60 years.
- It is thought to be caused by an autoimmune process.
- The most commonly affected joints are the fingers, thumbs, wrists, feet and ankles.
- Treatment includes disease-modifying drugs to suppress inflammation, analgesia and surgery in severe cases.
- The figure below shows a simple diagram that you can use to illustrate rheumatoid arthritis to your patients.

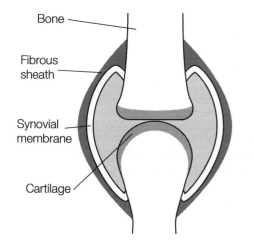
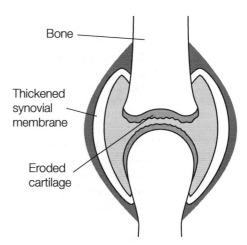

Data gathering

Open question
- *"Can you tell me more about your joint problems?"*

Focused/closed questions

HPC: *"Which joints are affected?"*

"When did the problems first start?" "Have the problems been getting worse?"

"Do you have any pain or swelling in the joints?"

"Any injury to your joints?"

"Is it worse at any particular time of the day?"

"Have you noticed any fever or weight loss or muscle pains?" (red flags)

"Have you had any eye or chest symptoms?"

FH: Any FH of rheumatoid arthritis?

DH: Are you currently taking any medication?

SH: Occupation? Who lives with you at home? *"Are you managing OK at home?"*

ICE: *"What concerns do you have about the joint pains?"*

"Does it stop you from doing the things you would normally be able to do?"

Examination:
- Joint examination.

Clinical management

Investigations
- Blood test – rheumatoid factor (present in two-thirds of people with RA), cyclic citrullinated peptide (CCP), CRP.
- X-ray.

Explanation to patient
- Arthritis means inflammation of the joints where two bones meet.
- In rheumatoid arthritis, the immune system makes antibodies against the tissues that surround each joint. This causes inflammation around the affected joint, and the cartilage which lines the joint can become eroded. Over time, this joint damage causes deformities of the joints.
- The main symptoms are pain and stiffness of the affected joints, and this is usually worse in the morning.

Management
- In people with newly diagnosed active rheumatoid arthritis, offer a combination of DMARDs plus short term glucocorticoids as first line treatment as soon as possible, ideally within 3 months of the onset of persistent symptoms (*NICE*, 2009, *CG79: Rheumatoid arthritis*).

Rheumatology/musculoskeletal

- NSAIDs and analgesia.
- Steroids, e.g. prednisolone, for flare-ups.
- Physical activity.
- Physiotherapy +/- occupational therapy.
- Safety net – return to GP if symptoms not improving.
- Referral to rheumatologist if suspected persistent synovitis of unknown cause or if poor response to initial management.

Role play

Information for doctor	Additional information for role player
Patient: Mrs AF *Age*: 70 years *SH*: Lives alone in 1 bed house with no carers. *FH*: Mother and grandmother had RA *PMH*: TIA 2007; hypercholesterolaemia *DH*: Simvastatin 40 mg OD, aspirin 75 mg OD *Information*: Recently saw practice nurse for influenza vaccination. You are a GP Registrar.	*PC*: *"I've been getting a lot of pain in my hands, and I'm struggling a bit".* *HPC*: Worsening pain for the past few months. Also stiffness worse in the morning. Right thumb and index fingers are the worst affected. No trauma. No muscle pains, fever or eye symptoms. *ICE*: **Difficulty at home especially with cooking and cleaning. Would like some extra help.** *O/E*: Swelling and deformity of both hands, especially right hand.

Tennis elbow

- Otherwise known as lateral epicondylitis, it is due to inflammation of the tendons around the elbow.
- Most commonly seen in the 30–50 year age group.
- Causes pain on the lateral side of the elbow, which often improves with rest, pain relief and/or physiotherapy.

Data gathering

Open question
- *"Can you tell me more about the elbow pain you have been experiencing?"*

Focused/closed questions
HPC: *"Where exactly are you experiencing the pain?" "Does the pain radiate?"*
"When did the pain start?"
"Is the pain present all the time or does it come and go?"
"Do you know what might have triggered the pain?"
"Have you tried any treatments so far?"
"Any swelling of the elbow?"
"Any fever?" (red flag)

SH: Occupation? Smoking/alcohol/illicit drug history? *"Do you play any sports regularly?"*

ICE: *"What were you hoping we might be able to do to help?"*
"Has the pain stopped you from doing anything that you would usually do?"

Examination: • Elbow examination (see *Appendix 1*).

Clinical management

Investigations
- Initially clinical diagnosis.
- If not improving consider MRI scan.

Explanation to patient
- Tennis elbow occurs due to inflammation of the tissue (the tendons) that connects the muscle to the bone at the elbow.
- It causes pain in the outer part of the elbow, and it is often worse with twisting movements of the arm (e.g. opening a jar).
- The pain is often caused by an injury to one or more of the tendons around the elbow. The injuries are often caused by overuse of the forearm , particularly seen in manual workers and racquet sports players.

Management
- Rest or modifying activities that bring on the symptoms.
- Analgesia (e.g. paracetamol, NSAIDs, codeine phosphate).
- Steroid injection.
- Physiotherapy.
- Elbow support or splint.
- Safety net – return to GP if above measures not helping.
- Referral for surgery (to remove the damaged part of the tendon).

Role play

Information for doctor	Additional information for role player
Patient: Mr PS *Age:* 37 years *SH:* Married with one child. Joiner. Non-smoker, 5 units alcohol/week. *FH:* Nil *PMH:* Arthroscopy of left knee 2008 *Information:* You are a salaried GP.	*PC:* *"I have been having trouble with my right elbow".* *HPC:* Pain in the right elbow for the past month. Pain mainly on the lateral side. Intermittent pain. **Worse when working.** Has tried paracetamol and Nurofen but no improvement. Slight swelling of the elbow. *ICE:* **Would like to know what is causing it, and would like some stronger painkillers.** *O/E:* Afebrile. Tenderness over right lateral epicondyle. Pain worse on supination of the right arm.

Carpal tunnel syndrome

- Pain and/or numbness of the hand, as a result of compression of the median nerve as it passes through the carpal tunnel at the wrist.
- A ligament called the retinaculum lies across the front of the wrist, and the carpal tunnel is the space between this ligament and the bones of the wrist.
- The figure below shows a simple diagram that you can use to illustrate carpal tunnel syndrome to your patients.
- Management includes analgesia, wrist splint, steroid injection or surgery.

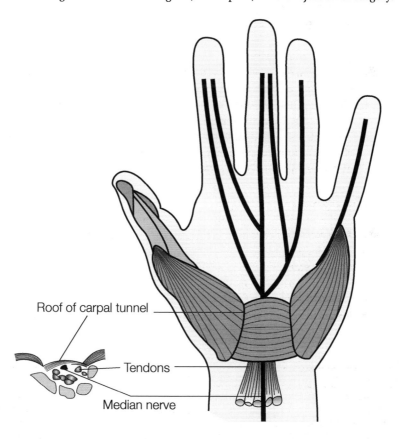

Roof of carpal tunnel

Tendons

Median nerve

Data gathering

Open question
- *"Can you tell me about the problem with your hand?"*

Focused/closed questions

HPC: *"When did the problem first start?"*

"Do you have any pain, numbness, burning, tingling or weakness in your hand?"

"Which fingers are specifically affected?"

"Are the symptoms worse at any particular time of the day?"

"Are you aware of any aggravating or relieving factors?"

"Have you noticed any wasting of your hand muscles?" (red flag)

"Did you injure your hand?"

PMH: Any history of arthritis or wrist problems? Any history of thyroid problems or diabetes? Are you pregnant?

FH: Any family history of carpal tunnel syndrome?

SH: Occupation? Manual work? Smoking/alcohol/illicit drug history?

ICE: *"What do you think is causing your symptoms?"*

Examination:
- Examination of the hand – check for muscle wasting, tenderness, power and sensation.
- Phalen's test – press the back of the hands together, flexing the wrists. The test is positive if the patient experiences tingling or increased numbness within 1 minute.
- Tinel's test – tap or press on the median nerve at the wrist. The test is positive if you experience tingling or a shock-like sensation.

Clinical management

Investigation
- FBC, U&Es, TFTs, CRP, ESR, fasting glucose (to check for possible causes).
- Nerve conduction studies or USS wrist (not routinely done).

Explanation to patient
- Carpal tunnel syndrome is caused by pressure on a nerve around the wrist.
- The nerve involved is the median nerve which supplies sensation to the thumb, index and middle fingers, and half of the ring finger. It also controls some of the movements of the thumb.

Management
- Leave alone – often resolves without any treatment. Return to GP if no improvement.
- Conservative management – weight loss, avoid over-use of the wrist.
- Wrist splint.
- Steroid injection – reduces inflammation.
- Surgery – the ligament is cut to ease the pressure on the carpal tunnel.
- If thenar wasting the patient must be referred to orthopaedics.

Role play

Information for doctor	Additional information for role player
Patient: Mrs RJ	*PC*: Tingling in left hand and painful left wrist.
Age: 78 years	*HPC*: Two month history but symptoms worsening.
SH: Lives alone, widowed, retired	**No trauma.** Numbness of left thumb, index and
PMH: Rheumatoid arthritis	middle finger. Worse at the end of the day.
DH: Naproxen	*ICE*: Worried about cause of tingling. **Restricts day**
Information: Last consultation 1 month ago due to	**to day tasks – pain when opening jars, etc.**
arthritic pain. You are a GP partner.	*O/E*: Numbness in lateral three digits. Tinel's test
	positive.

Dermatology

Eczema

- Atopic eczema describes a chronic inflammatory itchy skin condition which usually develops in early childhood.
- Typically the skin becomes dry and inflamed.
- The cause is not fully known, although it is thought that the oily barrier of the skin is reduced, making the skin more susceptible to irritants and allergens.
- Approximately 2 in 3 children with atopic eczema grow out of it by mid teens.
- The most commonly affected areas are the skin creases and around the neck. The face is commonly affected in babies.
- Treatments include emollients and topical steroids for flare-ups.

Data gathering

Open question
- *"What problems have you been experiencing with your skin?"*

Focused/closed questions

HPC: *"When did you first develop problems with your skin?"*
"How often do you get flare-ups?"
"Does your skin get dry and/or itchy?"
"Which areas of your skin are affected?"
"Do you have any infected and/or weepy areas?"
"Have you noticed any blistering of your skin?" (red flag)
"Do you have any painful areas of skin?" (red flag)
"Have you had any fever?" (red flag)
"Have you had any joint pains?"
"Are you aware of any particular triggers, for example, certain foods?"
"Any concerns with growth and development?" (child)

FH: Any FH of eczema, hayfever or asthma?

ICE: *"What were you hoping we could do to help with your skin?"*
"How has it been affecting you?"

Examination: • Skin examination.

Clinical management

Investigations

- No specific investigations.

Explanation to patient

- Eczema is inflammation of the skin which is often dry and itchy and it can flare up from time to time.
- Sometimes the inflamed areas can become weepy and infected.
- The cause is not fully known although it does run in families and it is also thought to be caused by a problem with the immune system.

Management

- Patient education including written information.
- Avoid using soaps and bubble baths as they can be skin irritants.
- Avoid scratching and wear cotton clothing.
- Antihistamines or crotamiton cream to reduce the itching (not routinely recommended, however).
- Use non-biological detergents.
- In bottle-fed infants under 6 months try eliminating cows' milk products.
- Emollients.
- Topical steroids for short term use for flare-ups.
- Antibiotics either topically or orally for infected eczema.
- Safety net – return if not improving.
- If suspected eczema herpeticum refer immediately to hospital (areas of rapidly worsening, painful eczema, with blisters or ulcerated lesions and possible fever).
- Routine dermatology referral if uncertain diagnosis, poor response to treatment, or if associated with severe or recurrent infections (*NICE*, 2007, *CG57: Atopic eczema in children*).

Role play

Information for doctor	Additional information for role player
Patient: Ms SM *Age*: 17 years *SH*: College student, lives with parents *PMH*: Eczema *DH*: Cetraben emollient cream, hydrocortisone cream BD/PRN for flare-ups *Information*: You are a locum GP.	*PC*: Flare-up of eczema in the last few days, which isn't settling with emollients and hydrocortisone. Dry, itchy skin on back of knees, hands and arms. **No weeping or blistering. No fever.** *FH*: **Sister and mum have eczema and asthma.** *ICE*: Would like some other cream to control the eczema. *O/E*: Scaly, red, inflamed patches especially on popliteal fossa and hands.

Psoriasis

- Skin condition that typically results in plaques of red, scaly skin.
- There are different types of psoriasis, but plaque psoriasis is the commonest type.
- Other types include scalp, nail, guttate, flexural, pustular or erythrodermic psoriasis.
- There is no cure, but treatments include emollients, vitamin D based creams, coal tar preparations, dithranol and steroid creams.

Data gathering

Open question
- *"Can you tell me more about the skin problems you are having?"*

Focused/closed questions

HPC: *"Where specifically have you got the skin problem?"*
"When did it develop?" "How has it progressed?"
"Have you tried any treatments so far?"
"Is your skin itchy?" "Is your skin painful or sore?"
"Have you noticed any nail or scalp changes?"
"Any pain in your joints?"

PMH: Any previous skin problems? Any medical conditions? Any recent illness?

FH: Any family history of psoriasis?

SH: Smoking/alcohol/illicit drug history? Occupation? Stress?

DH: Are you on any medications?

ICE: *"What do you think is causing this skin rash?"*

Examination:
- Skin examination including nails and scalp.
- Joint examination if joint symptoms from the history.

Clinical management

Investigations
- No specific investigations recommended.
- Occasionally a skin biopsy is done.

Explanation to patient
- Psoriasis is a skin condition that occurs because there is a faster turnover of skin cells than usual. This results in a build up of cells on the top layer of skin, which causes plaques to form. It is not clearly understood why this occurs. There is also some skin inflammation that occurs.
- Aggravating factors include stress, infections, drugs, smoking, sunlight and injury to the skin.

- Some people with psoriasis will also get joint and nail problems.
- Psoriasis can flare up from time to time and there is no definite cure.

Management

- Emollients – softens hardened plaques.
- Vitamin D based creams (calcipitriol, calcitriol) – reduce the rate of cell division of the skin cells.
- Coal tar – reduces turnover of the skin cells and reduces inflammation. Can be used for plaque psoriasis or for scalp psoriasis in combination with salicylic acid preparations.
- Dithranol – reduces plaque formation.
- Steroid creams – reduce inflammation.
- If poor response to the above treatments refer to dermatologist for consideration of PUVA (ultraviolet light treatment) or other specialist treatments.

Role play

Information for doctor	Additional information for role player
Patient: Mr JS *Age*: 40 years *SH*: Married with 2 children. Builder. Smokes 20 cigs/day. *PMH*: Nil *DH*: Nil *Information*: No previous consultations. You are a locum GP.	*PC*: "*I have had a problem with my skin for the past month*". *HPC*: Dry itchy skin, mainly on the elbows. Improved when I went on holiday to Spain last week but still present. **No painful joints. No scalp or nail changes.** *FH*: Father has psoriasis. *ICE*: Thinks it may also be psoriasis. Would like some cream to get rid of it as looks unsightly. *O/E*: Erythematous plaques on both elbows.

Acne

- Common cause of skin problems, especially amongst teenagers.
- Usually affects the face, but can also affect the back, neck and chest.
- Treatment includes topical preparations, retinoids, antibiotics or the combined oral contraceptive pill.

Data gathering

Open question

- *"Can you describe the problems that you have been having with your skin?"*

Focused/closed questions

HPC: *"How long have you had the acne for?" "Is it getting worse?"*
"Have you noticed any triggers for the acne?"

          "Have you tried any over the counter treatments?"

          "Do you have acne on other parts of your body?"

FH: Does anyone else in the family have acne or any other skin problems?

SH   Smoking/alcohol/illicit drug history? Occupation?

DH: Are you taking any other medications? (steroids, lithium and anti-convulsants can worsen acne)

ICE: *"How does your skin problem affect you?"* *"How does it affect your self esteem?"*

Examination: • Skin examination.

Clinical management

Investigations

- Nothing specific.

Explanation to patient

- Acne is caused by a problem with the glands beneath the skin that make sebum (oil).
- Some pores become blocked and the sebum becomes trapped. This can result in bacteria multiplying in these blocked pores. Inflammation can then occur in the surrounding skin.

Management

- Avoid any possible triggers or aggravating factors, e.g. cosmetic products or certain drugs.
- Topical preparations, e.g. benzoyl peroxide, retinoids (e.g. adapalene), antibiotics.
- Antibiotic tablets, e.g. tetracycline, lymecycline.
- Oral contraceptive pill, e.g. dianette.
- Referral to specialist if poor response to treatment or in severe cases of acne.

Role play

Information for doctor		Additional information for role player
Patient:	Mr TW	*PC*: Acne.
Age:	16 years	*HPC*: Acne not improving with medication given. No known triggers. Has spots on face and back.
PMH:	Nil	*SH*: Lives with parents and younger sister.
DH:	Benzoyl peroxide	*ICE*: **Feels self-conscious about his skin. Starting**
FH:	Nil	**college soon and keen to get problem sorted.**
Information:	Last consultation with GP 3 months ago – problem with acne. You are a salaried GP.	*O/E*: Moderate pustular and nodular acne on the face and back.

Endocrinology

Diabetes

- Diabetes mellitus is a long-term condition which occurs when the level of glucose in the blood becomes higher than normal.
- There are two main types of diabetes mellitus – type 1 and type 2.
- In type 1 diabetes the beta cells in the pancreas stop producing insulin, and the blood glucose level increases.
- In type 2 diabetes you still make insulin, but either you do not make enough for your body's needs or the cells in your body are unable to use this insulin properly.

Data gathering

Open question

- *"Can you tell me more about your symptoms and when it all started?"*

Focused/closed questions

HPC: *"Have you got any increased thirst or are you passing urine more than usual?"*
"Do you have any tiredness or weight loss?"
"Have these symptoms been getting worse?"
"Have you suffered with recurrent thrush or other infections?"
"Have you noticed any problems with your vision?"
"Do you have any problems with the sensation in your feet?"
"Any problems with chest pain?"
"Any vomiting, problems breathing or confusion?" (red flags – DKA/HONK)

FH: Any family history of diabetes?

PMH: Do you have any other medical conditions, e.g. hypothyroidism?

DH: Do you take any regular medications? Diuretics?

SH: Smoking/alcohol/illicit drug history? Occupation? Do you drive? Diet/exercise?

ICE: *"What do you think is causing these symptoms?"*

Examination:
- BP, pulse, respiratory rate.
- BMI.
- Visual acuity/fundoscopy.
- Foot examination.

Clinical management

Investigations
- Urinalysis – check for glucose, ketones and microalbuminuria.
- Bloods – fasting blood glucose, HbA1C, FBC, U&Es.

Explanation to patient
- Normally, the amount of sugar in the blood is controlled by a hormone called insulin, which is produced by the pancreas.
- When food is digested and enters the bloodstream, insulin moves any glucose out of the blood and into cells, where it is broken down to produce energy.
- In people with diabetes mellitus, the body is unable to break down glucose into energy because there is not enough insulin or the insulin doesn't work properly. If the glucose remains poorly controlled, this can result in various problems including eye, feet, and kidney problems, and there is an increased risk of developing heart disease or stroke.

Management (based on *NICE, 2009, CG66: Type 2 diabetes*)
- Refer to A&E immediately if any signs of DKA or HONK (glycosuria or ketonuria with tachycardia, hypotension, dehydration or altered level of consciousness).
- Monitor HbA1C every 2–6 months (aim for below 6.5%).
- Healthy diet – high fibre, low glycaemic index sources of carbohydrate. Low fat dairy products and oily fish. Control intake of saturated fats.
- Exercise, weight control, smoking cessation.
- Self-monitor plasma glucose for those on insulin, oral hypoglycaemics or to monitor changes during intercurrent illness.
- BP control (aim for <140/80 mmHg or <130/80 mmHg if kidney, eye or cerebrovascular damage):
  - Lifestyle advice – low salt diet, exercise.
  - ACE inhibitor – first line (use calcium channel blocker if chance of patient becoming pregnant)
  - Calcium channel blocker or diuretic – second line.
  - Monitor BP 6 monthly (or annually if no treatment required).
- Annual eye, foot and kidney function checks (or more frequently if any abnormalities detected).
- Lipid management:
  - Aim for total cholesterol <4.0 mmol/l and LDL <2.0 mmol/l.
  - Offer simvastatin 40 mg if >40 years and type 2 diabetic.
  - Offer fibrate if raised triglycerides not controlled with lifestyle changes or statin.
  - If target cholesterol still not reached, increase simvastatin to 80 mg or try another statin or ezetimibe.
- Offer low dose aspirin if >50 years or <50 years with other CV risk factors.
- Patient education programme and/or support group.

Type 1 diabetes
- Insulin.

- Referral to specialist diabetic nurse or endocrinologist at diagnosis.
- Aim for pre-prandial blood glucose level of 4–7 mmol/l and post-prandial level of <9 mmol/l.

Type 2 diabetes
- Diet, weight control and exercise.
- If HbA1C still ≥6.5% start metformin (introduce slowly to minimize GI side effects; also monitor U&Es & LFTs).
- If HbA1C still ≥6.5% add a sulfonylurea, e.g. gliclazide (beware of risk of hypoglycaemia).
- Consider substituting a DPP-4 inhibitor or thiazolidinedione for the sulfonylurea if a sulfonylurea is not tolerated.
- If HbA1C ≥7.5% add insulin (a thiazolidinedione can be added instead or exenatide if BMI ≥35).

Role play

Information for doctor		Additional information for role player	
Patient:	Mr JH	*PC*:	*"I was asked to come in to discuss my blood test results".*
Age:	50 years		
PMH:	Hypercholesterolaemia, hypertension	*HPC*:	**No polydipsia/polyuria/tiredness/weight loss.** No visual problems. No problems with sensation in the feet. **Enjoys sugary cakes.**
DH:	Simvastatin 40 mg, Coracten 30 mg OD		
FH:	Father has diabetes		
Information:	You are a GP Partner. This patient had a recent blood test: fasting glucose 8 (NR: 3–6)	*ICE*:	No concerns. Not sure why he was asked to come today. Feels fine.
		O/E:	NAD

Hypothyroidism

- Under-active thyroid gland, resulting in a decreased production of thyroxine.
- Common symptoms include tiredness, weight gain, constipation, dry skin and menorrhagia.
- Treatment is by replacing the decreased thyroid hormone with a medication called levothyroxine.

Data gathering

Open questions
- *"Your recent blood test has shown that you have an underactive thyroid gland. What do you know about hypothyroidism?"*
- *"What symptoms have you been experiencing?"*

Focused/closed questions
HPC: *"Has your weight changed recently?"*

> *"Have you been more tired than usual?"*
> *"Have you noticed any changes with your skin or hair?"*
> *"Any bowel symptoms?"*
> *"Any changes to your periods?"*
> *"Have you been feeling low in mood lately?"*

FH: Any family history of thyroid problems or other conditions?

SH: Who lives with you at home? Smoking/alcohol/drug history? Occupation?

DH: Do you take any regular medications?

ICE: *"What concerns you about these symptoms?"*

Examination:
- BP.
- Thyroid examination.
- Reflexes.

Clinical management

Investigations
- Thyroid function tests.

Explanation to patient
- Thyroxine is a hormone produced by the thyroid gland in the neck. It helps to control the body's metabolism. In hypothyroidism the thyroid gland doesn't made enough thyroxine and so the body's functions slow down. It is important that this is treated to avoid complications such as heart disease from developing.
- After starting on levothyroxine you will need to have regular thyroid function blood tests to check that the level of medication is sufficient.

Management
- Levothyroxine starting dose usually 50 mcg daily (patients receive free NHS prescriptions).
- Check TFTs 1–3 monthly until stable and then annually thereafter.
- Safety net – if symptoms not improving return to GP.

Role play

Information for doctor	Additional information for role player

Patient: Mrs SO
Age: 42 years
PMH: NIDDM
DH: Metformin, gliclazide
SH: Smokes 10 cigs/day, 2 units alcohol/week. Receptionist.
Information: Recent blood test:
  • serum TSH: 7 (NR: 0.35–4.94)
  • serum T$_4$: 2 (NR: 9–19)
  • serum T$_3$ 4.5 (NR: 4–8.3)
You are a salaried GP.
	PC: "*I have come in to discuss my blood test results*".
	HPC: Has been feeling more tired than usual. Thought it was likely stress at work. **Some weight gain also. No bowel symptoms. No skin changes. No increased thirst or polyuria.** No low mood.
	ICE: Thinks she might be anaemic.
	O/E: BMI – 28. Thyroid examination – NAD. HR – 52.

Hyperthyroidism

- 'Overactive' thyroid gland resulting in raised levels of thyroid hormone in the bloodstream.
- Commonest cause is Graves' disease.
- Symptoms include weight loss, palpitations, tremor, restlessness and thyroid swelling.
- Management includes medication, radio-iodine treatment or surgery.

Data gathering

Open questions
- *"Can you tell me more about the symptoms you have been experiencing?"*
- *"Can you tell me more about the neck swelling you have developed?"*

Focused/closed questions

HPC: *"Have you noticed any weight loss, tremor, palpitations or diarrhoea?"*
"Any irritability, anxiety or changes in your energy levels?"
"Any neck swelling or eye changes?"

FH: Any family history of thyroid problems?

DH: Are you taking any regular medications?

SH: Alcohol/smoking/illicit drug history? Occupation? Caffeine intake?

ICE: *"What concerns you about these symptoms?"*

Examination:
- BP, pulse.
- Thyroid examination.
- Cardiac examination.

Clinical management

Investigations
- TFTs.
- Ultrasound scan of thyroid gland if palpable thyroid mass.

Explanation to patient
- Thyroxine is a hormone made by the thyroid gland which controls the metabolism of the body.
- In hyperthyroidism there is an overactive thyroid gland which results in an increased production of thyroxine. This results in a faster metabolism.
- With treatment the outlook is good.

Management (based on *NHS CKS*, 2008, *Hyperthyroidism*)
- Carbimazole or propylthiouracil under specialist advice only.
- Consider prescribing a beta-blocker (e.g. propranolol) if the patient has a tremor or tachycardia.

- Radio-iodine (by specialist only).
- Surgery – involves removing part of the thyroid gland.
- Follow-up – regular thyroid function tests. If symptoms worsen to return to GP.
- Admit to hospital if severe signs and symptoms of hyperthyroidism, e.g. fever, agitation, heart failure, confusion or if the patient is systemically unwell.

Role play

Information for doctor	Additional information for role player
Patient: Ms AR *Age*: 32 years *SH*: Accountant, lives with partner. No alcohol/smoking/illicit drugs. *FH*: Nil *PMH*: Migraine *DH*: Nil *Information*: No recent consultations. You are a salaried GP.	*PC*: Weight loss, tremor, palpitations. *HPC*: Palpitations and tremor for past month. Heart beat feels fast but regular. Noticed slight neck swelling. Lost 5 kg in the past month. No visual symptoms. *ICE*: **Worried about her heart.** *O/E*: HR 100 bpm. Heart sounds I + II + 0. Thyroid swelling in the neck, no AF. No eye signs.

Tired all the time

- Very common presentation in general practice.
- Approximately 50% of cases will have a psychological cause.
- Only 20–30% cases will have an identifiable physical cause.
- Differential diagnoses include depression, obstructive sleep apnoea, treatment with a sedative drug, chronic fatigue syndrome, anaemia, diabetes and thyroid disease.

Data gathering

Open questions
- *"Can you tell me more about the tiredness you've been experiencing?"*
- *"What exactly do you mean by feeling tired all the time?"*

Focused/closed questions
HPC: *"When did the problem first start?"*

"Have you identified any possible triggers for the tiredness?"

"Is the problem getting worse?"

"What were your previous levels of energy like, and how does this compare with the present?"

"When do you usually go to bed, and what time do you wake up?" "Any daytime napping?"

"Have you noticed any other changes, for example, weight changes, passing more urine than normal, increased thirst, sleep disturbance, skin changes or bowel problems?"

"Any changes in your mood?"

PMH: Any significant medical problems?

DH: Are you taking any medications? Beta-blockers? Sleeping tablets?

FH: Anyone in the family with any similar problems or any illnesses that run in the family?

SH: Alcohol/smoking/illicit drug history? Occupation? Stress?

ICE: *"Do you have any idea why you might be feeling tired all the time?"*

Examination:
- BMI.
- Check for signs of anaemia.
- Thyroid examination – if any symptoms in the history.
- PHQ-9 questionnaire – if any symptoms of depression.

Clinical management

Investigations
- Urinalysis – to check glucose.
- FBC – to check for anaemia.
- TFTs – to check for hypothyroidism.
- U&Es – to exclude any renal problems.
- CRP, ESR and monospot test for glandular fever.

Explanation to patient
- Tiredness is a very common problem, and we will try to eliminate any medical cause for the tiredness, for example, anaemia or an underactive thyroid.
- The management will depend on the cause of the tiredness.

Management
- Sleep hygiene – avoid napping in the day, reduce caffeine and alcohol, increase exercise.
- If iron deficiency anaemia – ferrous sulphate.
- If hypothyroidism – start levothyroxine.
- If depression, consider self help or anti-depressants.
- Safety net – see GP again if not improving.

Role play

Information for doctor	Additional information for role player
Patient: Mr AC *Age*: 38 years *SH*: Social worker who lives with partner. *FH*: Mother and sister – depression. *PMH*: Asthma *DH*: Salbutamol, beclomethasone *Information*: You are a GP Partner. This patient was seen by your colleague 1 week ago due to tiredness. Was sent for blood tests: • Hb 15 g/dl (NR: 13–18) • ferritin 120 ng/ml (NR: 30–400) • serum TSH 0.65 mIU/l (NR: 0.35–4.94) • serum T$_4$ 12 pmol/l (NR: 9–19) • Na 140 mmol/l (NR: 136–145) • K 4.5mmol/l (NR: 3.5–5.1) • urea 4 mmol/l (NR: 2.5–8) • creatinine 80 mmol/l (NR: 64–111)	*PC*: *"I am feeling tired all the time and have come for my blood test results".* *HPC*: Tiredness for the past few months. **Feels a bit low in mood. Stress at work.** Not sleeping very well – wakes up very early and has difficulty getting to sleep. **Concentration at work poor.** No weight changes. No bowel or urinary symptoms. Previously quite energetic. *ICE*: Worried about what is causing the tiredness. Would like a referral if no other cause is found. *O/E*: BMI 22; PHQ-9 score 16/27 (moderate–severe depression).

Chronic fatigue syndrome

- A condition involving a complex range of symptoms that includes fatigue, malaise, headaches, sleep disturbance, difficulties with concentration and muscle aches.
- Also known as ME (myalgic encephalomyelitis).
- A diagnosis should be made after excluding other possible diagnoses, and after symptoms have persisted for at least 4 months in an adult (3 months in a child).
- Usually develops between 20 and 45 years of age and is more common in females.
- Symptoms can last for years, although the outlook for young people is more optimistic.

Data gathering

Open question
- *"Can you tell me more about the fatigue you have been experiencing?"*

Focused/closed questions
HPC: *"When did your symptoms first start?"*
"How often do you feel tired/fatigued?"
"Does this tiredness limit the activities that you do?"
"How would you describe your concentration?"
"What is your sleep pattern like?"
"Do you suffer with any headaches or muscle pains?"

"Any recent weight loss or breathing problems?" (red flag)
"Any changes to your mood?"

SH: Occupation? Who lives with you at home? Smoking/alcohol/illicit drug history?

ICE: *"How is this affecting your day to day life?"*

Examination (to exclude other causes):

- Check temperature and look for signs of anaemia.
- Lymph nodes.
- Throat.
- Abdominal examination – check for hepatomegaly or splenomegaly.
- Mental state examination (see *Appendix 3*).

Clinical management

Investigations

- Urinalysis for protein, blood and glucose.
- Blood tests for FBC, U&Es, TFTs, LFTs, ESR, CRP, random blood glucose, CK, calcium, coeliac antibodies.

Explanation to patient

- Chronic fatigue syndrome is a condition resulting in long term disabling tiredness. It can also cause problems with sleep, muscle pains and/or headaches.
- The cause is not known, although it may be caused by a viral infection.
- There are no tests to prove that you have chronic fatigue syndrome, and there is no specific cure. Certain treatments can ease symptoms.

Management (based on *NICE, 2007, CG53: Chronic fatigue syndrome/Myalgic encephalomyelitis*)

- Sleep hygiene and offer relaxation techniques.
- Introduce rest periods.
- Regular well balanced diet.
- Graded exercise therapy – gradual, progressive increase in physical activity/exercise.
- Cognitive behavioural therapy.
- Offer help through occupational health services and disability services. If possible, advise flexible adjustments to work rather than stopping altogether.
- Occupational therapy or physiotherapy if required.
- Offer information about local and national self-help and support groups.
- Offer referral to specialist within 6 months of presentation if mild CFS or 3–4 months if moderate symptoms (NICE).
- Consider offering a low dose TCA for poor sleep or pain – but not if the person is already taking an SSRI (NICE).
- Regularly review management plan every 4–6 weeks and advise to return sooner if symptoms not improving or worsening.

Role play

Information for doctor	Additional information for role player
Patient: Mrs KS *Age*: 32 years *SH*: Lives with husband. Works as teacher. *PMH*: Nil *DH*: Nil *FH*: Mother has chronic fatigue syndrome. *Information*: You are a GP Registrar.	*PC*: *"I feel so weak and have no energy".* *HPC*: Six month history of daily tiredness. Occasional muscle aches. Concentration generally poor. No weight loss. Doesn't feel able to work. Feels a bit fed up. *SH*: No alcohol/smoking/illicit drugs. *ICE*: **Thinks she might have 'ME' as her mum suffers with it and has similar symptoms. Would like a sick note (has been off work for 10 days).**

Drug and alcohol problems

Alcohol abuse

- In the UK, it is estimated that 24% of adults drink in a hazardous or harmful way (*NHS Information Centre*, 2009, *Statistics on alcohol* – www.ic.nhs.uk/statistics-and-data-collections/health-and-lifestyles/alcohol).
- Alcohol dependence is defined as a cluster of behavioural, cognitive and physiological factors that typically include a strong desire to drink alcohol, and difficulties in controlling its use (DSM-IV definition by American Psychiatric Association).
- Alcohol-related problems include Wernicke's encephalopathy, liver disease and acute and chronic pancreatitis.
- Management includes help from local alcohol services and a detoxification programme.

Data gathering

Open question
- *"Can you tell me more about your alcohol problem?"*

Focused/closed questions

HPC: *"How much alcohol are you drinking each day?"*
"What exactly are you drinking?"
"Why have you decided to seek help now?"
"Has anyone been concerned about your drinking?"
"Do you get annoyed at people who comment on your drinking?"
"Do you feel guilty about your drinking?"
"Do you wake up in the morning and feel the need to have a drink of alcohol?"
"Do you have any abdominal pain?"
"Any problems with your balance?"
"Have you ever had any seizures?"
"Have you noticed any yellow discoloration of your skin?"

PMH: Any past problems with alcohol?

SH: Smoking/illicit drug history? Occupation? Who lives with you at home? Do you drive?

FH: Any FH of alcohol problems?

ICE: *"What help would you like with your drinking problem?"*

Examination: • BP.
- Focused examination including check for tremor, jaundice, spider naevi, and abdominal examination.

Clinical management

Investigations
- Bloods – FBC, B$_{12}$, folate, LFTs, GGT.
- Liver ultrasound scan if abnormal LFTs.

Explanation to patient
- It is very important that you cut down on your drinking, as persistent drinking at harmful levels can result in damage to almost every organ or system of the body.

Management
- Advise patient to contact local alcohol services, e.g. Alcoholics Anonymous.
- Vitamins – vitamin B co-strong 30 mg daily, thiamine 200–300 mg daily.
- Detoxification – benzodiazepines such as chlordiazepoxide and diazepam are used in UK clinical practice for the management of alcohol-related withdrawal symptoms (*NICE, 2010, CG100: Alcohol-use disorders: physical complications*).
- Consider acamprosate and/or disulfiram for those who wish to abstain from alcohol (*SIGN, 2003, 74: Management of harmful drinking and alcohol dependence in primary care*).
- If any symptoms/signs of delirium tremens (tremor, confusion, fits, visual hallucinations), or if at high risk of alcohol withdrawal seizures, refer urgently to hospital for medically assisted withdrawal (*NICE, 2010, CG100: Alcohol-use disorders: physical complications*).
- Offer social support – sick note, benefits, employment, housing, DVLA, etc.
- Regularly review every few days during period of withdrawal or abstinence and safety net – return to GP or go to A&E if any seizures, problems with withdrawal or symptoms of Wernicke's delirium tremens as described above.

Role play

Information for doctor	Additional information for role player
Patient: Mrs PP	*PC*: Drinking problem.
Age: 52 years	*HPC*: Came to discuss drinking problem. Has been drinking 2 bottles of wine each night for the past couple of months since separating from husband. Concerned about her drinking.
SH: Recently separated from husband, lives with 2 children. Housewife.	
PMH: Nil	**Doesn't drive.**
DH: Nil	*SH*: No illicit drug use, non-smoker
Information: Last appointment was with salaried GP 6 months ago due to marital problems. You are a GP Partner.	*ICE*: **Worried as husband has been physically abusive. Sister also very concerned about her drinking and wants to take the children away from her.**
	O/E: Abdominal exam NAD, BP 145/90.

Opiate addiction

- Opiate addiction is a disorder of the central nervous system that arises from continuous use of opiates.
- There is a growing problem of dependency on opiate drugs, for example, prescription drugs such as morphine and codeine and non-prescription drugs such as heroin.
- Signs of excessive opiate use include sedation, euphoria, respiratory depression, small pupils, nausea, vomiting, slurred speech and confusion.
- Abrupt or sudden withdrawal of these drugs induces a withdrawal syndrome which includes symptoms of insomnia, irritability, vomiting, depression and muscle pain.

Data gathering

Open question

- *"Can you tell me more about your drug addiction problem?"*

Focused/closed questions

HPC *"How long have you had the addiction for?"*
"Have you ever injected drugs?" "If so, have you ever shared needles?"
"Have you ever tried to get help for this problem before?" "If so, what happened?"
"Do you have any problems with your sleep or your mood?"
"Any vomiting, irritability or muscle aches?" (red flags)
"Any thoughts of self harm?"
"Have you experienced any hallucinations?"
"Do you have any chest pain or shortness of breath?" (red flags)
"How is your mood?"

PMH: Any previous history of drug/alcohol problems?
Any past psychiatric history?
Any history of Hep B/C/HIV?

SH: Who lives with you at home? How is this problem impacting on other family members? Occupation? Finances? Smoking/alcohol?

ICE: *"What help would you like for your drug dependency?"*

Examination: • Pulse, BP.
- Check injection sites for signs of infection if IV drug user.

Clinical management

Investigations

- ECG if concerned about heart rate/rhythm.
- Urine drug screen.
- Hep B/C, HIV testing.

Explanation to patient

- After prolonged opiate drug use, the nerve cells in the brain, which would otherwise produce natural painkillers (known as endorphins), cease to function normally. The body stops producing endorphins because it is receiving opiates instead. The degeneration of these nerve cells causes a physical dependency to opiate drugs.

Management

- Hepatitis B vaccination if IV drug user.
- Needle exchange programme if continuing to use IV drugs.
- Self-help/support groups – local drug services.
- Detoxification programme – methadone or buprenorphine should be offered as first line treatment in opioid detoxification (*NICE*, 2007, *CG52: Drug misuse: opioid detoxification*).
- Assess personal, social and mental health needs (*NICE*, 2007, *CG52: Drug misuse: opioid detoxification*) – housing, benefits, DVLA, etc.
- Offer CBT or psychodynamic therapy for people who have co-morbid depression and anxiety disorders (*NICE*, 2007, *CG52: Drug misuse: opioid detoxification*).
- Review patient on a weekly basis and ask them to return sooner if any new or worsening symptoms.

Role play

Information for doctor	Additional information for role player
Patient: Mr JE *Age*: 38 years *SH*: Unemployed, lives alone in a council flat. Smokes 20 cigs/day, drinks 20 units alcohol/wk. *PMH*: Nil *Information*: You are a locum GP.	*PC*: *"I would like help to get clean from drugs".* *HPC*: Currently heroin user – injects. Has been using IV drugs for the past 2 years. Doesn't share needles. Also occasional cannabis use. **Has had Hep B vaccine. Been tested for HIV/Hep B/C – negative.** Has difficulty sleeping. Feels low. Has financial problems also. *ICE*: Would like to start on a methadone programme. Never tried to quit before. *O/E*: Pulse and BP normal. No infected injection sites.

Appendix 1

Clinical examinations

Focused cardiovascular examination

- Expose the patient appropriately (ask permission first).
- Position the patient correctly (ideally at 45°).
- Inspection – pallor, cyanosis, scars, oedema, clubbing, JVP.
- Palpation – pulses (rate, rhythm), BP, apex beat, heaves, thrills.
- Auscultation – apex and carotid area (more detailed auscultation required if murmur heard). Listen to lung bases.

Focused respiratory examination

- Expose the patient appropriately (ask permission first).
- Position the patient at 45° ideally.
- Inspection – check hands for clubbing and peripheral cyanosis. Check tongue for pallor/cyanosis. Check respiratory rate and check chest for scars.
- Palpation – check for position of trachea and chest expansion. Check for cervical lymphadenopathy.
- Percussion – front and back of chest ideally.
- Auscultation – listen at front and back.

Focused gastrointestinal examination

- Expose the patient appropriately (ask permission first).
- Lie the patient flat if possible, with arms to the side.
- Inspection – check for jaundice, pallor, spider naevi or gynaecomastia. Check hands for clubbing, cyanosis, palmar erythema or Dupuytren's contracture. Check abdomen for distended veins or masses.
- Palpation – check for cervical lymphadenopathy. Palpate each area of the abdomen then palpate liver, spleen, kidneys and bladder (or focus depending on history).
- Percussion – liver, spleen and for shifting dullness if relevant.
- Auscultation – check for presence and quality of bowel sounds.

Neurological examination

Cranial nerves

I	Olfactory	Have you noticed any change in your sense of smell or taste?
II	Optic	Any problems with your vision? If so, check visual acuity with Snellen chart. Also check visual fields. Fundoscopy.
III	Occulomotor	Accommodation, visual movements, direct/consensual light reflex.
IV	Trochlear	As for occulomotor tests.
V	Abducens	Same as occulomotor and trochlear tests.
VI	Trigeminal	Check sensation on both sides of the face and compare (branches of trigeminal nerve).
VII	Facial	Raise eyebrows, clench teeth, blow cheeks out, close eyes tightly and stop me from opening them.
VIII	Vestibulo- cochlear	Check gross hearing by whispering in each ear. If any concerns with hearing perform Rinne's and Weber's tests.
IX	Glosso-pharyngeal	Taste sensation as above.
X	Vagal	Say 'aaaagghh' (look for deviation of the uvula).
XI	Accessory	Please can you shrug your shoulders? Check power in sternocleidomastoid muscles by moving neck side to side against resistance.
XII	Hypoglossal	Can you stick your tongue out? (check for deviation, atrophy and fasciculations).

Whispered speech test

- See www.youtube.com/watch?v=dsS7d6_k1F8 to watch examination being carried out.
- To make a basic assessment of a patient's hearing, you need to mask the non-test ear by blocking it with your finger, and then ask them to repeat random numbers that you speak into the test ear.
- You can start with a whisper, and if they are unable to hear this then increase the volume in incremental steps.

Rinne's test

- Strike a 512 Hz tuning fork and place the fork behind the ear, firmly on the mastoid process.
- Then hold the vibrating fork a few inches away in front of the ear.
- In a normal ear, the patient should hear the tuning fork louder in front of the ear than behind.
- If a patient has a conductive hearing loss, they will hear the bone conduction behind the ear louder than the air conduction.

Weber's test

- Strike a 512 Hz tuning fork and place the base of the fork on the patient's forehead.
- A patient with normal hearing should hear the sound equally on both sides.
- If a patient has unilateral conductive hearing loss, the sound will localise to the affected ear.
- If a patient has unilateral sensorineural loss, the sound will localise to the opposite ear.

Thyroid examination

- Hands – check pulse, check for tremor.
- Eyes – check for exophthalmos and lid lag.
- Neck – inspect, check swallowing and tongue protrusion, palpate neck for mass, percuss neck swelling, auscultate for bruits.
- Check reflexes.

Shoulder examination

- Expose both shoulders (ask permission first).
- Look – from front, side and rear inspecting for scars, erythema, muscle wasting, asymmetry, swelling and any deformity of the shoulder joint.
- Feel – check temperature, palpate bony landmarks, joint line and surrounding muscles for any tenderness, crepitus or effusions.
- Move – check active/passive movements of abduction/adduction, flexion/extension, internal/external rotation.
- Function – arms behind head and scratching back.

Knee examination

- See www.youtube.com/watch?v=fNUGyNYVhqE to watch examination being carried out.
- Look – inspect the patient lying and standing for any scars, swelling, erythema, deformity (e.g. varus/valgus) or muscle wasting around the knee.
- Feel – palpate the medial and lateral joint line with the knee flexed. Then with the knee extended palpate the patella and the popliteal fossa. Check for effusion using a patellar tap and then check temperature on both sides.
- Move – check active/passive flexion/extension.
- Anterior draw test – tests for stability of anterior cruciate ligament.
- Lachman's test – tests for stability of anterior cruciate ligament.
- Function – assess gait.

Elbow examination

- See www.youtube.com/watch?v=bMJjbIT3zek&NR=1&feature=fvwp to watch examination being carried out.
- Look – from front, side and back, looking at the carrying angle and for any flexion deformity, scars, swelling, rheumatoid nodules, etc.

- Feel – check temperature and palpate the olecranon and lateral/medial epicondyles for tenderness.
- Move – flexion, extension, pronation and supination (active and passive).
- Function – e.g. put hand to mouth.

Back examination

- Look – from behind inspect for deformity (lordosis/scoliosis/kyphosis), bruising, swelling, muscle wasting, asymmetry.
- Feel – check temperature, palpate spinal processes, sacro-iliac joint and para-spinal muscles for tenderness.
- Move – flexion, extension, lateral flexion, hip rotation, straight leg raise.
- Limb reflexes and sensation.

Diabetic foot examination

- Inspection – gait, ulcers, deformity, erythema, swelling.
- Palpation – foot pulses, temperature, capillary refill.
- Sensation – soft touch, pinprick, vibration, proprioception, temperature.
- Motor – check range of movement of foot.

Neurological motor and sensory examination

(see www.patient.co.uk for further details)

- Observation – involuntary movements, muscle symmetry, atrophy & gait.
- Tone – ask the patient to relax. Flex and extend wrists, elbows, knees and ankles. Observe for increased or decreased tone. Check for clonus also.
- Power – ask the patient to move against your resistance. Always compare one side to the other. Grade the power based on the MRC scale 0–5. Test upper and lower limbs.
- Reflexes – biceps, triceps, knee, ankle and wrist.
- Check plantar response (Babinski).
- Co-ordination – heel/shin and finger–nose test.
- Sensation – close eyes, compare symmetrical areas of the body. Check light touch first, and can continue with other modalities if any abnormalities detected.

Appendix 2

Sexual history

- Firstly explain that you are going to ask a few sensitive questions that are important in order to find out more about the problem.
- Ensure that the patient is relaxed and don't be judgemental.
- Privacy and assurance of confidentiality are also important.

Questions to ask

- *"When did you last have sexual intercourse?"*
- *"Was it with a regular partner or a casual partner?"*
- *"Was your partner male or female?"*
- *"Did you have vaginal sex, oral sex or anal sex?"*
- *"Did you use a condom?"*
- *"Have you had any other sexual partners in the past 3 months?"* If so, repeat the questions as above.
- *"Have you had any previous STIs?"*
- Females: *"When was your last menstrual period?" "Do you use regular contraception?" "If so, what?" "When was your last cervical smear?" "Any previous abnormal smear tests?"*
- HIV/Hep B/Hep C risk assessment: *"Have you ever paid for sex?" "Any sexual partners from high risk countries such as Thailand or sub-Saharan African countries?" "Have you or your partner ever injected drugs?" "Have you ever been vaccinated against hepatitis B?"*

Additional questions to ask those under 16 years

- *"How old is your partner?"*
- *"Was the sex consensual or did you feel coerced/forced?"*
- *"Are your parents/carer aware of your sexual activity?"*
- *"Are your parents/carer aware of your attendance here today?"*
- *"Do you feel able to tell your parents/carer?"*
- *"Have you ever been drunk or under the influence of drugs when having sexual intercourse?"*
- Any history of depression or other mental health problems?

N.B. Where children under the age of 13 report sexual activity, this should be discussed, in confidence, with a local child protection lead. Reporting to social services and the police may be appropriate but is not mandatory.

Appendix 3

Mental state examination

The following should be observed and commented on:
- **Appearance and behaviour** – patient's self care, eye contact, gait, and whether the patient is agitated, hostile or has abnormal movements.
- **Speech** – rate, volume and pressure of speech. Also note whether any incoherence, neologisms or mutism.
- **Mood** – patient's mood subjectively and objectively.
- **Thought** – content of thoughts and form (flight of ideas, thought block, etc.)
- **Perception** – any hallucinations (e.g. visual or auditory) or delusions?
- **Insight** – does the patient have any insight into their illness/mental state?

Abbreviated mental state examination

The following questions should be asked to a patient to assess cognition/memory (total score out of 10):
1. Age
2. Time
3. Address – remember 42 West Street (for recall later)
4. Year
5. Name of current location
6. Identification of two people
7. Date of birth
8. Year of World War I
9. Present monarch
10. Count out 20 down to 1
11. Recall address from earlier